Fat Burning
Exercise & Diet

FAT BURNING

Exercise & Diet

Johannes Roschinsky

Meyer & Meyer Sport

Original title: Fatburning – Workout, Ausdauer, Ernährung
© Aachen: Meyer & Meyer, 2003
Translated by Heather Ross

British Library Cataloguing in Publication Data
A catalogue record for this book is available from the British Library

Fat Burning – Exercise & Diet
Johannes Roschinsky
Oxford: Meyer & Meyer Sport (UK) Ltd., 2004
ISBN 1-84126-140-8

© 2004 by Meyer & Meyer Sport (UK) Ltd.
Aachen, Adelaide, Auckland, Budapest, Graz, Johannesburg,
Miami, Olten (CH), Oxford, Singapore, Toronto
Member of the World
Sports Publishers' Association (WSPA)
www.w-s-p-a.org
Printed and bound by: Gráficas Santamaría, Spain
ISBN 1-84126-140-8
E-Mail: verlag@m-m-sports.com
www.m-m-sports.com

CONTENTS

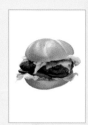

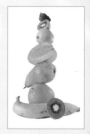

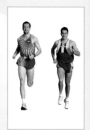

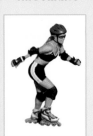

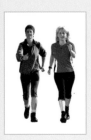

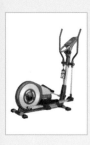

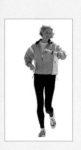

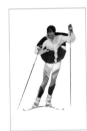

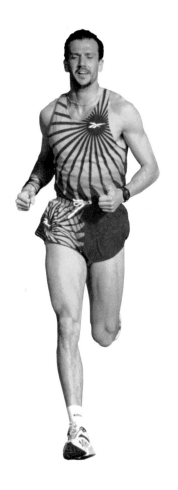

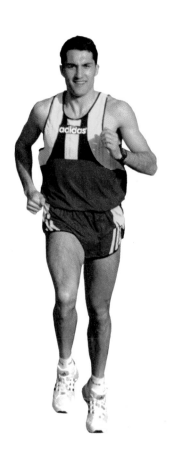

Foreword

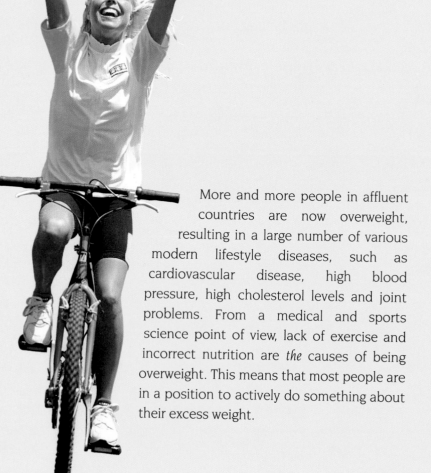

More and more people in affluent countries are now overweight, resulting in a large number of various modern lifestyle diseases, such as cardiovascular disease, high blood pressure, high cholesterol levels and joint problems. From a medical and sports science point of view, lack of exercise and incorrect nutrition are *the* causes of being overweight. This means that most people are in a position to actively do something about their excess weight.

This book is not an advanced work on diet or running. It includes the general theoretical principles of *body weight* and *nutrition*, the detailed description of various endurance sports and relevant training tips, it is a comprehensive introduction for all those who want to lose weight by eating healthily and exercising regularly.

This book would not have been possible without other people's help. I would therefore like to thank the following Marketing/Production managers: Oliver Guetzlaff (Kettler), Dr Harald Beitat (Polar) and Reinhard Hetzender (Loeffler). Others who deserve my thanks are Michael Marx, head of the company Dega Sport and Dr. Dieter Hackfort, head of the Sports Psychology and Sports Pedagogy department of the Munich Military University.

My colleagues Hans-Bernd Übbing and Ralf Kriegel deserve special thanks for critical remarks and constructive suggestions. Grateful thanks to the companies Polar, Kettler, K2, Technica, MPK and Engelberg-Titlis Tourismus AG for their valuable support in the preparation phase of the book.

I hope that this book helps you to both to find the right endurance sport for you and, by combining it with a sensible and healthy diet, to attain your ideal weight. On this note, I hope you enjoy reading this book and have fun training.

Johannes Roschinsky
Spring 2004

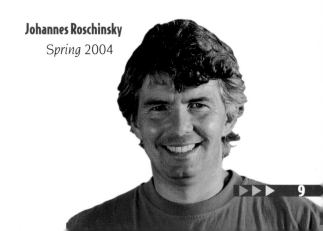

CHAPTER 1

Introduction

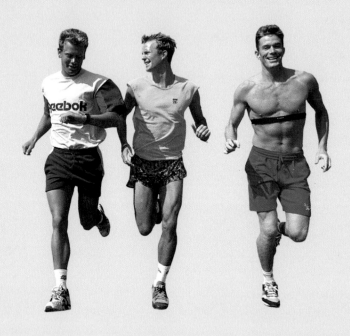

Almost every adult, and a high percentage of young people, has already tried to lose weight, i.e. to burn fat, without much success in most cases. Ignorance of the optimal fat-burning techniques, lack of success and the resulting rapid abandonment of the set goals just reinforces the vicious circle effect for many people. The mistaken belief that one's ideal weight can be achieved and maintained with a on-off crash diet will not go away (Yo-yo effect). The number of calories consumed during exercise is also still over-estimated by most people.

The recipe should be: change nutrition *and* exercise habits. Those who want to keep weight off should not unilaterally either do physical activity or change their eating habits.

Only a combination of qualitatively and quantitatively correct nutrition and regular exercise lead to the desired long-term result. Endurance sport plays an important role, as most people can reach a loading duration of more than half an hour relatively quickly by increasing the loading volume, and thereby stimulating the fat metabolism (adipolysis) more and more.

In general, mental factors, such as stress, loneliness, depression and frustration, should not be neglected as they affect nutritional (comfort eating) and exercise (laziness and low motivation) behavior, thereby obstructing a planned weight reduction.

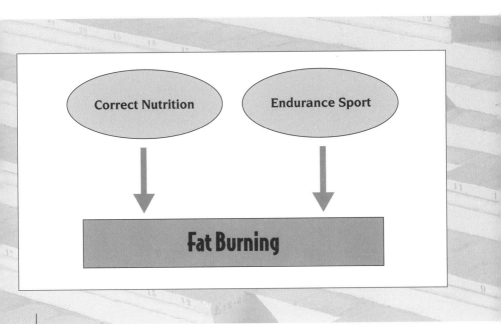

Figure 1: The two pillars of fat burning

The Health Risks of Obesity

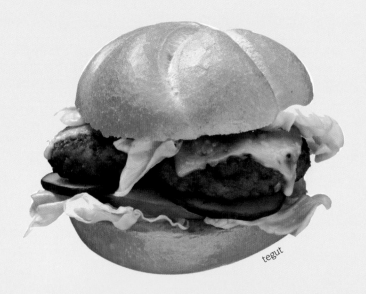

tegut

The World Health Organization (WHO) defines obesity as the biggest chronic health problem. In most industrialized countries, more than a third of adults and a quarter of children are now overweight. The consequential costs for the health service reach billions annually. The causes and consequences of obesity are extremely complex.

2.1 Causes of Obesity

Obesity often has quite differing causes, whereby, in most cases, several aspects interact and mutually strengthen each other. Everyday stress, genetic defects and illnesses also figure alongside incorrect nutrition and lack of exercise as the most important causes of obesity.

Incorrect Nutrition, Lack of Exercise and Everyday Stress

Incorrect nutrition, lack of exercise and everyday stress (e.g., work, loneliness, depression) are significant causes of obesity. If the causes lie in nutrition or in lack of exercise, then with the right motivation, the individual can lose weight relatively easily. This book will describe in detail the various ways to do this.

Genetic Defects and Illnesses

It is more difficult if the cause is genetic and if certain illnesses are involved. We are also talking here about pathological obesity (morbid adiposity). This topic will only be covered superficially here and should be left to the corresponding medical technical literature.

Genetically caused obesity is usually the result of several gene defects (polygenetic causes). In the meantime, we can assume that in the origin of obesity with corresponding genetic disposition, various genes are involved. Obesity can thereby develop in adulthood or childhood. Finally, even in this case, the overweight adult is still the result of genotype (genetic disposition) and their environment (fatty food).

Some illnesses, like hypothyroidism, Cushing Syndrome or brain tumors can also lead to obesity.

Hypothyroidism is caused by the production of too little or no thyroid hormones (thyroxin and triodthyronin). It causes all metabolic processes in the body to slow down considerably.

This underfunction requires lifelong medicinal treatment with an artificial metabolic hormone (Levothyroxin). With proper dosage, there are almost no side-effects.

Cushing's Syndrome is a hormonal disorder caused by the overproduction of cortisol, a hormone from the adrenal glands and also by the long-term use of cortisone. Cushing's Syndrome is a rare disease with many possible consequences (among others, weight gain, skin changes, raised blood pressure, muscle weakness, osteoporosis, depression, diabetes).

The consequences of the increase in cortisol as a disease were first described in 1909 by the American brain surgeon Harvey Cushing, who gave his name to it. Cortisol is formed in the adrenal glands and is one of the most important hormones in the body. Without it, death is inevitable.

The most frequent cause of Cushing's Syndrome is the long-term therapeutic use of high doses of cortisone (i.e., for bronchial asthma, rheumatic diseases and chronic inflammable stomach disorders).

After successful therapy, in many cases, cortisone can be reduced gradually. This eventually gets rid of Cushing's Syndrome. If Cushing's Syndrome has occurred without the use of cortisone, a dysfunction in the pituitary gland or the adrenal glands is likely. Pituitary gland or adrenal gland tumors can also cause Cushing's Syndrome.

2.2 Consequences of Obesity

Like the causes, the consequences of obesity are many and varied. Obesity initially combines most of them with negative mental, physiological and orthopedic consequences.

The psychosocial consequences are no less important, and, for many people, are harder to deal with. Extreme obesity is often seen to be linked to low self-confidence, low self-esteem and often also with a reduction in sexual attractiveness.

In addition, physical performance is reduced by obesity, and, from an orthopedic point of view, the entire supporting and musculoskeletal system is placed under considerably greater pressure, resulting in spinal and joint problems, especially in the lower limbs.

Extreme obesity often leads to a high resting pulse rate, arteriosclerosis, increased risk of heart attack, gout and constipation among other things. Women can encounter problems during pregnancy and when giving birth.

Obesity increases blood volume and chronically overloads the mostly also out-of-condition heart. With further resulting diseases, obesity forms the so-called deathly quartet, also known as *metabolic syndrome*.

This represents the following four of the five main risk factors (smoking is the fifth) for heart attack, which, in combination, reduce life-expectancy:

▶ FAT BURNING

- ▶ Obesity
- ▶ Diabetes mellitus (with increased insulin production)
- ▶ Increased blood lipid concentration (particularly triglycerides)
- ▶ High blood pressure

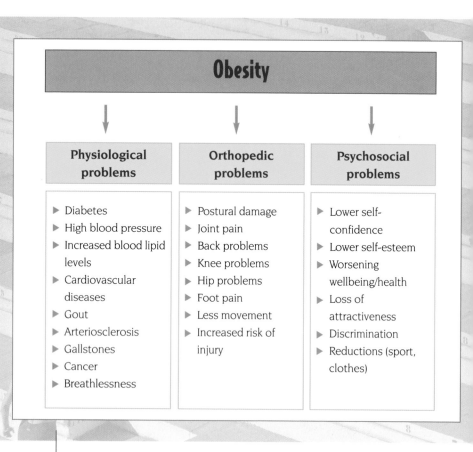

Obesity		
Physiological problems	**Orthopedic problems**	**Psychosocial problems**
▶ Diabetes ▶ High blood pressure ▶ Increased blood lipid levels ▶ Cardiovascular diseases ▶ Gout ▶ Arteriosclerosis ▶ Gallstones ▶ Cancer ▶ Breathlessness	▶ Postural damage ▶ Joint pain ▶ Back problems ▶ Knee problems ▶ Hip problems ▶ Foot pain ▶ Less movement ▶ Increased risk of injury	▶ Lower self-confidence ▶ Lower self-esteem ▶ Worsening wellbeing/health ▶ Loss of attractiveness ▶ Discrimination ▶ Reductions (sport, clothes)

Figure 2: The most important consequences of obesity

2.3 Weight Measurement

The best time to weigh yourself is in the morning before getting dressed and having breakfast. There are many suggestions as to the most accurate way of classifying one's measured weight, as in the end everyone wants to know if they are underweight, overweight or normal.

Two popular methods are the Broca formula and the Body Mass Index (BMI). Both serve as guidelines for an adult of normal weight. The weight tables of the US-based Metropolitan Life Insurance Co. appear to be even more suitable, as they take gender, height and build into account.

The oft-recommended "feel-good weight" has the advantage that individual well-being is not dictated by figures. There are actually no strict regulations on body weight and nutrition. The disadvantage, however, is that one cannot simply trust one's intuition, as these days, most peoples' exercise and eating habits are incorrect.

Individual factors, such as genetic conditions, physical activity (someone with a large muscle mass weighs more than someone without), and nutritional education in childhood (certainly the formation of fat cells), can affect weight. The figures calculated in all methods should be interpreted accordingly.

From this point of view, the terms *overweight* and *obesity* are in most cases used as synonyms. This is, strictly speaking, not correct, as the term *overweight* is initially only meant as above normal body weight. *Obesity*, on the other hand, occurs when the proportion of body fat in the whole body is clearly increased. So, bodybuilders or strength athletes (weight lifters, shot putters), for instance, often have both a high body weight and a low proportion of fat. For this reason, everyone who wants to reduce their body fat should not only measure their weight at regular intervals, but also their body fat.

Broca Formula

Familiar formulae for calculating weight are only indicative. For many years, the most popular formula for calculating normal weight has been the Broca formula. It was developed in the 19th century by the French doctor Pierre Broca. While carrying out medical research on soldiers, he noticed that the average weight was approximately a person's height minus 100. From this, he developed a formula for normal weight:

Height (cm) – 100 = normal weight

Criticisms of the Broca formula on the part of food scientists are firstly that gender-specific differences are not taken into account. Also, that the body weight arrived at in this way is too high for most people. In addition, it should be noted that the Broca formula works best for average body weights. The particularities of different body frames are also not taken into account.

A modified Broca formula provides a much better benchmark and also takes into account gender-specific differences. So, for women, the ideal weight is 15% below normal weight, due to their higher proportion of fat; and for men, the ideal weight is 10% below the normal weight due to their heavier build. This gives two formulae for the calculation of ideal body weight:

> Women: height (cm) – 100) – 15% = ideal weight
> Men: (height (cm) – 100) – 10% = ideal weight

Body Mass Index (BMI)

A better basis for calculation for body weight is the Body Mass Index (BMI). This is calculated in a non-gender-specific way as follows:

> Body weight (kg) : height (m²) = Body Mass Index

The resulting value is compared with the norm values.

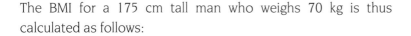

Below 18:	underweight
18-25:	normal weight
26-30:	slightly overweight
Over 30:	very overweight

The BMI for a 175 cm tall man who weighs 70 kg is thus calculated as follows:

> 70 : (1.75 x 1.75) = 22.857

The Body Mass Index of the person is rounded up to 22.9, meaning that his weight is normal.

The BMI is better suited to the evaluation of body weight than the Broca formula. From a nutritional science point of view, a BMI of 20-25 for men and of 19-24 for women is desirable and corresponds to normal weight. Values up to 30 correspond to overweight and above 30 to fat (obese).

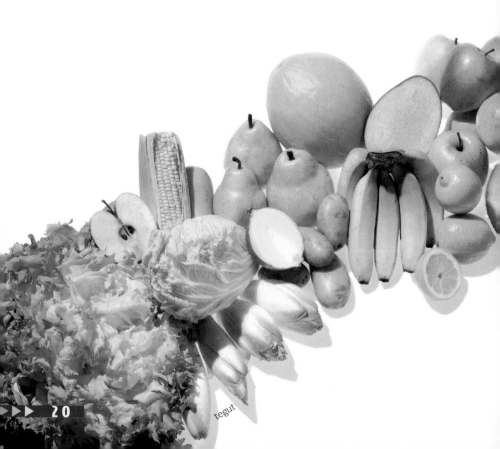

tegut

Table 1: BMI values for men and women

	Women	Men
Underweight	< 19	< 20
Normal Weight	19 – 24	20 - 25
Overweight Grade I (slightly overweight)	24 - 30	25 - 30
Overweight Grade II (Obese)	30 - 40	30 –40
Overweight Grade III (Extremely obese)	> 40	> 40

The BMI for normal weight shifts upward a little with age:

Table 2: Age-dependent BMI

Age	BMI – Normal weight
19 – 24	19 - 24
25 – 34	20 - 25
35 – 44	21 - 26
45 – 54	22 – 27
55 – 64	23 – 28
> 65	24 – 29

Metropolitan Life - Height and Weight Tables

The weight tables of the US Metropolitan Life Insurance Co. take into account gender, height and build. There are clear differences in the latter due to such factors as genetics (big bones) or physical training (a large muscle mass makes one heavier than otherwise). The features of each respective build and gender are dealt with optimally in the following tables. The normal weight range for each category is also relatively wide.

For example, the normal weight for a 1.68 m tall woman with medium frame can lie between 59 and 65 kg. If we compare extremes, e.g., two 1.68 m tall women, one with small bone structure and the other with a heavy physique, the normal weight range increases to 54 – 72 kg.

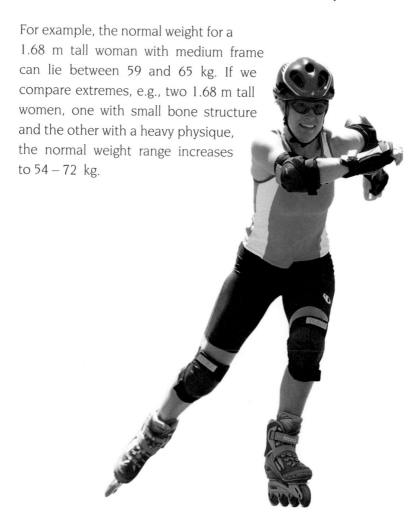

Table 3: Metropolitan Life – Height/Weight tables for women (in kilograms)

Height(cm)	Small Frame	Medium Frame	Large Frame
147	46-50	49-55	54-59
150	47-51	50-56	54-61
152	47-52	51-57	55-62
155	48-54	52-59	57-63
157	49-55	54-60	58-65
160	50 - 56	55-61	59-67
163	52-58	56-63	61-68
165	53-59	58-64	62-70
168	54-60	59-65	63-72
170	56-62	60-67	65-74
173	57-63	62-68	66-76
175	59-64	63-69	68-77
178	60-66	64-71	69-78
180	61-67	66-72	70-80
183	63-68	67-73	72-81
185	64-70	68-75	73-83
188	65-71	70-76	74-84
191	67-73	71-78	76-85
193	68-74	73-79	77-87

Table 4: Metropolitan Life – Height/Weight tables for men (in kilograms)

Height(cm)	Small Frame	Medium Frame	Large Frame
157	58-61	59-64	63-68
160	59-62	60-65	63-69
163	60-63	61-66	64-71
165	61-63	62-67	65-73
168	62-64	63-68	66-74
170	63-66	64-70	68-76
173	63-67	66-71	69-78
175	64-68	67-73	70 80
178	65-70	68-74	72-82
180	66-71	70-75	73-83
183	68-73	71-77	74-85
185	69-74	73-79	76-87
188	70-76	74-81	78-89
191	72-78	76-83	80-92
193	73-80	78-85	82-94
196	75-82	79-87	84-96
198	77-83	81-89	87-98
201	79-85	83-92	89-101
203	81-87	85-94	91-103
206	83-89	87-96	93-105
208	84-91	88-98	96-107
211	86-93	90-101	98-110

2.4 Body Fat Measurement

The first reaction of people who want to lose weight is to jump on the scales. Few of them know that it is not absolute body weight but rather the percentage of body fat that is important in fat burning. Only the body fat percentage accurately reflects a person's current body composition, nutritional status and personal fitness.

A crash diet mostly involves only the loss of water and muscle mass. In extreme cases, this even makes the body fat percentage rise. A high body fat percentage also carries an increased risk of cardiovascular disease, diabetes and certain types of cancer, as well as a guaranteed reduction in mental and physical fitness.

By regularly monitoring body fat, one can very quickly see the first signs of success. This has a motivational effect and helps get over potentially difficult periods. Systematic body fat reduction with a combined nutrition and exercise program can only be monitored by regular measurement of body fat. The reduction of the body fat percentage with the simultaneous increase in muscle mass are the real signs of success of a fat burning program.

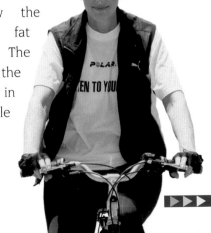

The two tables below show the recommended maximum body fat percentage for men and women. The values result from a study by the Institute for Aerobics Research in Dallas from 1994, with a total sample of 16,936 people.

Table 5: Body fat percentage in women

Age	Women			
	Excellent	Good	Average	Bad
20-24	**18,9**	22,1	25,0	29,6
25-29	**18,9**	22,0	25,4	29,8
30-34	**19,7**	22,7	26,4	30,5
35-39	**21,0**	24,0	27,7	31,5
40-44	**22,6**	25,6	29,3	32,8
45-49	**24,3**	27,3	30,9	34,1
50-54	**25,8**	28,9	32,3	35,5
55-59	**27,0**	30,2	33,5	36,7
> 60	**27,6**	30,9	34,2	37,7

Table 6: Body fat percentage in men

Age	Men			
	Excellent	Good	Average	Bad
20-24	10,8	14,9	19,0	23,3
25-29	12,8	16,5	20,3	24,3
30-34	14,5	18,0	21,5	25,2
35-39	16,1	19,3	22,6	26,1
40-44	17,5	20,5	23,6	26,9
45-49	18,6	21,5	24,5	27,6
50-54	19,5	22,3	25,2	28,3
55-59	20,0	22,9	25,9	28,9
> 60	20,3	23,4	26,4	29,5

There are a variety of ways of measuring body composition. If you regularly weigh yourself and measure your body composition and still want to record your body fat level, here are a few tips to follow when measuring:

Tips

▶ Always take the measurement at the same time of day
▶ The conditions should always be comparable
▶ For example, always measure yourself in the morning before breakfast
▶ Always use the same equipment
▶ Check the accuracy of your equipment by measuring several times consecutively.

There are several ways of ascertaining body composition, ranging from complicated laboratory methods to simple home kits. Laboratory methods include:

▶ Computer tomography
▶ X-ray methods
▶ Densitometry (underwater weighing)

Simple, and more importantly, very cheap methods of body weight analysis that are described briefly below, include:

▶ Bio Impedance Analysis (BIA)/Body fat analysis scales
▶ Near infrared spectroscopy (Futrex®)
▶ Skin fold thickness measurement

Bio Impedance Analysis (BIA)/
Body Fat analytical Balance

Bio-electrical Impedance Analysis (BIA) is based on the differing conductivity of different types of tissue to an alternating current. Four electrodes are placed on the body, through which an alternating current of 500-800 μA at 50kHz passes, which penetrates extra- as well as intracellular fluid space. The person lies down as the measurement is carried out by two current-bearing electrodes in the center of the backs of the hands and soles of the feet. In other measuring systems, the person stands barefoot with the heels and forefeet each on an electrode, which are attached to the weighing platform of a set of scales. Although only the lower limbs are involved in the measuring process, it is possible to draw conclusions as to the composition of the whole body.

tegut

New equipment tries to take population-specific differences into account with different calculation formulae, whereby physical activity level is incorporated into the calculation. This is based on the observation of the larger carbohydrate reserves of trained people, which absorb extra body fluid. The reproducibility of the results of Bio-electrical Impedance Analysis depends on keeping certain conditions. As measurement is very strongly dependent on total body fluid, and on its distribution in the extra- and intracellular space disturbances in the body fluid content due to food or fluid consumption (especially alcohol), physical activity, diuretic consumption, blood donation, edema or during the female cycle lead to mistakes in the evaluation of body fat levels. The fullness of the bladder and the body temperature also affect measurement.

Near Infrared Light Spectroscopy

Near infrared measurement was introduced in 1984 by Conway, et al. It is based on the principles of light absorption, reflection and spectroscopy. This new technology was compared with others in various studies and, subsequently, a new measuring device was brought onto the market. It uses NIR energy (near infrared interactance).

The NIR method is based on the fact that light and heat rays are absorbed, reflected and dispersed at different wavelengths by substances. Different chemical compounds in the body, such as fat, protein, water, starch, sugar, etc., can be measured thanks to their differing absorption values, which depend on the different characteristic bindings of atoms in the constituent substances.

The devices of the only current manufacturer Futrex Inc., which owns the worldwide patent, comprise an input unit with microprocessor, a light beam and an optical standard. The unit of account consists of a clear control panel, an adequate LED display where the results appear and a thermo-transfer printer for the documentation of results.

Measuring is made by a light beam protected by a sleeve from other light interference. The rays from the infrared diodes penetrate up to 4 cm into the tissue and are reflected according to the type of tissue. The rays remaining after absorption are measured with a silicon sensor. This single-point measurement gives sufficient information on the total body fat percentage.

Skin Fold Thickness Measurement

Calipometry is a simple way of measuring body fat percentage. As about 50-70% of body fat tissue is stored subcutaneously, with the aid of a fat-measuring pincer (calipers), the skin fold thickness can be ascertained in different parts of the body.

The skin and subcutaneous fat are pressed between the thumb and index finger and lifted off the underlying muscles. The thickness of the skin fold produced is measured with the calipers. The body fat percentage can then be calculated using an algorithm of the varying skin fold thickness.

Apple or Pear Type?

The actual location of fat on the body is very important in determining the health risks of being overweight. It has been known for years that the distribution of fat over the body favors the onset of common diseases like diabetes and heart disease.

There are two types of fat distribution: the apple type and the pear type. As a rule of thumb, the health risks are higher for the apple type than for the pear type. The latter is more characteristic of women, whose fat is distributed mainly over the hips and thighs. Fat distribution over the abdominal area, characteristic of the apple type, is more typical of men.

The so-called *spare tire*, or the deposit of fat around the stomach or chest, constitutes a far greater danger for health than that around the hips and thighs. People who belong to the apple type suffer more frequently from high blood pressure, coronary heart disease, diabetes and metabolic disorders than people with a more pear-shaped fat distribution.

Body fat distribution is defined as the waist circumference divided by the hip circumference. Women with a proportion of up to 0.84 are classified as pear-shaped, above that is an apple type. For men, an apple figure begins with a waist-hip ratio of 1.0.

Test for body fat distribution
▶ Measure around your waist with a tape measure (at the level of your tummy button)
▶ Then measure your hip circumference
▶ Divide the waist circumference by the hip circumference

The value is optimal if:

▶ For women it is not more than 0.84
▶ For men it is not more than 1.0

2.5 Basal and active metabolic Rates

The energy requirement for one day is termed the total energy expenditure. This consists of the so-called basal rate and active rate. The daily energy expenditure is a very individual thing and is determined by age, height, gender, body weight, physical activity at work and the type and extent of leisure activity.

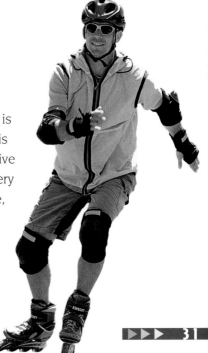

Basal Rate

Basal Rate means the amount of energy required by the body to maintain a temperature of 37° at rest and at room temperature. For this, the body needs about 25 calories (kcal) per kilogram of body weight per day. The basal metabolic rate of a person weighing 70 kg would therefore be: 70 x 25 = 1,750 kcal. The basal rate accounts for 50-70% of the total energy expenditure.

The basal rate amount depends firstly on the muscle mass, as the skeletal muscles are the body's biggest organ and where the lion's share of the energy is burnt. The basal metabolic rate also decreases with age, partly because muscle mass decreases, but also because many metabolic processes run more slowly with age and thus require less energy. Many people move less as they get older, thus reducing the movement-dependent energy requirement. This is one explanation for age-related weight gain.

Active Rate

The active rate is the amount of energy needed per day by our bodies to carry out work or recreational activities, or the energy we require for movement. The active metabolic rate is regulated by physical activity, heat production, digestion and the requirement for growth, pregnancy and lactation. Basal and active rates together give the total metabolic rate, i.e., the total energy expenditure per day.

Light physical activity can increase the basal rate by a third and heavy physical activity by more than two-thirds.

Strictly speaking, the nutrition-dependent *consumption metabolic rate* must be considered along with the basal and active rates.

This refers to the energy used by the body to make use of the food consumed, and constitutes about 6-10% of the total energy expenditure. Compared to the utilization of carbohydrates, for which the body requires relatively high amounts of energy, the body converts eaten fats into body fat with little energy expenditure. This emphasizes once again the problems of a fat-rich diet.

A targeted weight reduction will only be maintained by a negative energy balance of the calorie metabolism. So each person's body weight depends on their calorie intake, calorie consumption and genetic pre-conditions. As the latter are irreversible, our body weights can only be controlled by calorie intake (diet) and calorie consumption (the body's basal and active metabolic rate).

There are two possibilities:

▶ Reduction of calories by eating more sensibly (qualitative and quantitative)
▶ Increase energy consumption by additional exercise

The most successful way is undoubtedly a combination of regular aerobic exercise and a controlled and reduced-calorie diet.

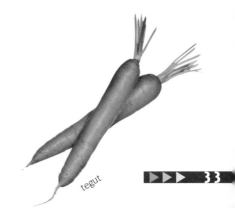

tegut

Correct Nutrition

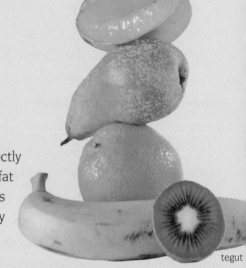

tegut

A healthy diet is directly relevant to the subject of fat burning and forms the basis of a sensible and healthy lifestyle.

Anyone who wants to lose weight should be familiar with the main features of a correct, needs-compatible diet to be able to help increase their quality of life.

The basic principles of a healthy diet are that it should be balanced, nutritionally and physiologically adequate and needs-compatible, i.e., appropriate for the body's active metabolic rate. This applies to the main nutrients, carbohydrates, proteins and fats, as well as vitamins, minerals, trace elements and the fluid balance.

3.1 Carbohydrates

Carbohydrates, along with fats and proteins, are the best nutritional energy providers. The ideal nutrient ratio to aim for is 55-60% energy demand from carbohydrates, 25-30% from fats and 10-15% from proteins.

Long-chain carbohydrates, the so-called *polysaccharides*, in the form of noodles, rice, potatoes, fruit and vegetables, should be the preferred type of carbohydrate. Short-chain carbohydrates (*monosaccharides*), in the form of sweets and glucose should be avoided as they only lead to a rapid increase in the blood sugar level and then a sharp energy drop.

3.2 Fats

Fats provide more than double the amount of calories (1g fat = 9kcal) as the same amount of carbohydrates or protein (1g = 4kcal). As most people's fat percentage of nutritional energy consumption is far too high at 35-45%, they excessively promote weight gain and considerably diminish their physical and mental ability. In a healthy diet, fat consumption should only constitute 25-30% of the nutritional energy consumed, of which 50% is from animal and 50% from vegetable fats.

Animal fats are mainly found in butter, lard and meat as saturated fatty acids, while vegetable fats can be found as unsaturated fatty acids in margarine and vegetable oils.

The World Health Organization (WHO) recommends a significant reduction in saturated fat consumption for most people, to protect against arteriosclerosis, especially of the coronary vessels.

Ideally, the amount of fat consumed should consist of a third each of unsaturated, saturated and polysaturated fats. The more "unsaturated" the fat, the more spreadable or liquid (oily) its consistency.

3.3 Protein

Proteins (Greek *protos* = *the first*) are the building blocks of the cells. Protein should make up 10-15% of nutritional energy consumption and, as for fats, be 50% of animal origin and 50% of vegetable origin.

The most important animal protein providers are milk, cheese, quark, eggs, fish and lean meat. Vegetable protein is mainly to be found in cereals, potatoes, pulses and cereal products (oats, pasta).

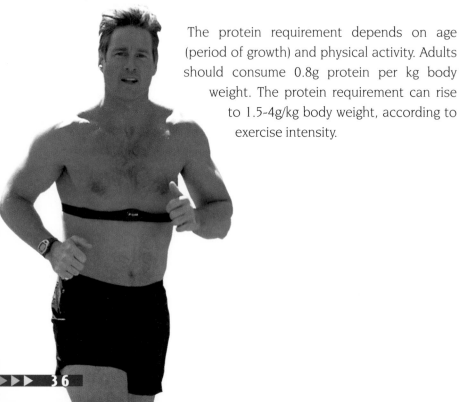

The protein requirement depends on age (period of growth) and physical activity. Adults should consume 0.8g protein per kg body weight. The protein requirement can rise to 1.5-4g/kg body weight, according to exercise intensity.

3.4 Vitamins, Minerals and Trace Elements

Vitamins, minerals and trace elements provide no energy in themselves, but are vital organic substances that must be included in our diet. They are involved in the control and regulation of metabolic processes and are particularly to be found in salads, vegetables, fruit, cereals and pulses.

When the body sweats during physical activity, it mainly loses minerals and trace elements, but also vitamins, e.g., vitamin C. A high exercise load can quickly treble the demand. That's why it is important to replace the deficit even during exercise with mineral water, fruit squashes and bananas; or before exercise to ensure that the above substances have been taken in sufficient quantities.

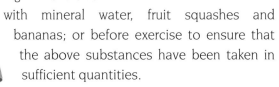

3.4.1 Vitamins

Vitamin (literally = *the stuff of life*) are complex organic compounds that are very effective, even in small quantities. They are just as essential for the body as proteins, carbohydrates and fats. The most important functions of vitamins are:

▶ Involved in nearly all functions of the body

▶ Helping the body utilize the food consumed

▶ Absorbing proteins, carbohydrates and fats from food

▶ Maintaining physical and mental efficiency

▶ Metabolising the body's own substances, such as hormones, enzymes and blood cells

▶ Regulating growth in adolescence

▶ Strengthening the body's defenses

▶ Stabilizing of the functioning of the nervous system

▶ Delivering energy and nutrients for tissues and organs

The body either forms vitamins in insufficient quantities or not at all, so they must be supplied by our food. They can be divided into fat-soluble or water-soluble vitamins. Vitamins A, D, E and K can only be absorbed by the body in combination with fats; a spoon of yogurt or sour cream is enough. Vitamin B_1, B_2, B_6, B_{12}, C, H and folic acid are water soluble though.

As the main source of vitamins is the diet, deficiencies and overdoses can occur. An overdose of water-soluble vitamins can usually be eliminated within the urine. An overdose of fat-soluble vitamins can lead to serious health problems, which are greatly underestimated:

▶ An overdose of vitamin A during pregnancy can lead to fetal abnormalities
▶ An overdose of vitamin D can lead to calcification of the arteries, bone deformities and kidney failure

Possible vitamin deficiency symptoms are illustrated in the following two tables.

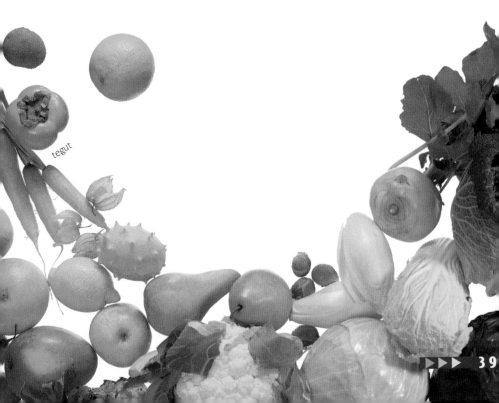

tegut

Table 7: The most important fat-soluble vitamins

Fat-soluble Vitamins				
Vitamin	Function	Deficiency Symptom	Food Sources	Daily Requirement
Vitamin A	▶ Eyesight ▶ Growth ▶ Reproduction	▶ Night blindness ▶ Weight loss ▶ Acrokeratosis ▶ Overdose produces serious health problems	▶ Cod liver oil ▶ Liver ▶ Mango ▶ Carrots ▶ Milk ▶ Egg yolk	▶ 0.8 mg (women) ▶ 1.0 mg (men) ▶ 1.5 mg (lactating)
Vitamin D	▶ Bone formation ▶ Cartilage formation	▶ Rickets ▶ Osteoporosis ▶ Bad teeth	▶ Liver fat ▶ Egg yolk ▶ Dairy products ▶ Fish	▶ 0.005 mg ▶ 0.01 mg (elderly)
Vitamin E	▶ Anti-inflammatory ▶ Anti-fatigue ▶ Delay of aging process ▶ Amblyiopia ▶ Tiredness ▶ Protection from carcinogenic substances	▶ Vitamin E deficiency very rare in healthy people	▶ Wheat germ oil ▶ Maize oil and soya oil ▶ Vegetables ▶ Almonds ▶ Leafy vegetables ▶ Eggs ▶ Liver	▶ 12 mg (women) ▶ 15 mg (men) ▶ 17 mg (lactating)
Vitamin K	▶ Blood clotting ▶ Prevents internal bleeding	▶ Slow blood clotting	▶ Spinach ▶ Kale ▶ Yogurt ▶ Eggs ▶ Liver	▶ 0.001 mg/kg body weight

Table 8: The most important water-soluble vitamins

		Water-soluble Vitamins		
Vitamin	Function	Deficiency Symptom	Food Sources	Daily Requirement
Vitamin B_1	▶ Growth ▶ Nerve function ▶ Mental efficiency	▶ Weight loss ▶ Loss of appetite ▶ Muscle weakness ▶ Mental instability ▶ Growth problems	▶ Wholemeal products ▶ Pork ▶ Liver ▶ Milk ▶ Potatoes ▶ Yeast	▶ 1.0 mg (women) ▶ 1.2 mg (men)
Vitamin B_2	▶ Eyesight ▶ Growth ▶ Reproduction ▶ Skin, nails, hair ▶ Energy metabolism	▶ Skin problems ▶ Stunted growth ▶ Nerve problems ▶ Anemia (in serious cases)	▶ Whole meal ▶ Pork ▶ Liver ▶ Milk ▶ Cheese ▶ Eggs	▶ 1.2 mg (women) ▶ 1.4 mg (men)
Vitamin B_6	▶ Protein metabolism ▶ Fat metabolism	▶ Skin damage ▶ Mouth and eye inflammations ▶ Nerve problems	▶ Yeast ▶ Eggs ▶ Kiwi ▶ Vegetables ▶ Milk ▶ Bran	▶ 1.2 mg (women) ▶ 1.5 mg (men) ▶ 1.9 mg (lactating)
Vitamin B_{12}	▶ Red blood cell production ▶ Protein metabolism ▶ Nerve function ▶ Memory	▶ Anemia ▶ Reduced cell division ▶ Protein synthesis problems	▶ Only in animal products (liver, fish, eggs, milk, cheese)	▶ 0.003 mg ▶ 0.004 mg (lactating)
Vitamin C	▶ Connective tissue ▶ Cartilage ▶ Wound healing process	▶ Susceptibility to infection ▶ Scurvy (very rare)	▶ Citrus fruits ▶ Berries ▶ Peppers ▶ Green vegetables ▶ Potatoes ▶ Liver	▶ 100 mg ▶ 150 mg (lactating)

Water-soluble Vitamins				
Vitamin	Function	Deficiency Symptom	Food Sources	Daily Requiremer
Vitamin H	▶ Skin, nails, hair ▶ Prevents premature greying	▶ Skin and mucous problems ▶ Hyperactivity	▶ Cauliflower ▶ Soy flour ▶ Liver	▶ 0.03-4 mg
Folic Acid	▶ Prevention of deformities ▶ Growth ▶ Nerve function ▶ Memory ▶ Skin ▶ Appetite	▶ Blood formation defects ▶ Inflammation of mucous ▶ Gastrointestinal problems	▶ Apricots ▶ Liver ▶ Meat ▶ Wheatgerm ▶ Pumpkin ▶ Avocado ▶ Beans ▶ Yeast	▶ 0.4 mg ▶ 0.6 mg (pregnant and lactating women)

tegut

3.4.2 Minerals

Minerals do not provide energy either, but are absolutely essential for our bodies. Minerals are required, even in small amounts, for all metabolic and building processes. Neither our nervous system nor our skeletal muscles can work without them.

An undersupply of minerals is usually avoided by a balanced diet with enough vegetables and wholegrain products. The danger of undersupply mainly occurs when food loses its mineral content during the preparation process.

Table 9: The most important minerals

Mineral	Function	Food Source
Mineral Sodium (Na)	▶ Stabilization of blood pressure ▶ Regulation of the pH balance ▶ Food uptake in the intestine ▶ High blood pressure on over-consumption ▶ Additional uptake only necessary after heavy sweating	▶ Sausage ▶ Cheese ▶ Tinned food ▶ Convenience foods
Potassium (K)	▶ Nerve function ▶ Muscle function ▶ Working of various enzymes ▶ Electrolyte balance	▶ Vegetables ▶ Pulses ▶ Bananas ▶ Spinach
Magnesium (Mg)	▶ Nerve function ▶ Muscle function ▶ Working of various enzymes	▶ Milk ▶ Fruit ▶ Poultry ▶ Soya beans ▶ Fish ▶ Vegetables
Calcium (Ca)	▶ Nerve impulse transmission ▶ Stabilization of cell membranes ▶ Bones and teeth ▶ Increased requirement during pregnancy ▶ Counteracts osteoporosis	▶ Milk ▶ Hard cheese ▶ Whole grain products ▶ Spinach ▶ Broccoli ▶ Green cabbage
Chloride (Cl)	▶ Maintenance of tissue tension ▶ Composition of stomach acidity	▶ Available with potassium in all salty food
Phosphorus (P)	▶ Energy supply to cells ▶ Bones and teeth ▶ Growth	▶ Milk ▶ Meat ▶ Fish ▶ Cola drinks ▶ Sausage ▶ Soft/processed cheese

3.4.3 Trace Elements

As well as vitamins and minerals, trace elements are vital for many physical functions (e.g., blood formation, growth). So, fluoride stabilizes our skeleton, strengthens our dental enamel and should repress microorganisms that are involved in the formation of caries.

Trace elements, as their name implies, are present in very small quantities in our bodies.

Table 10: The most important trace elements

Trace Elements	Function	Food Source
Iron (Fe)	▶ Blood formation ▶ Oxygen transport ▶ Increased requirement during pregnancy, adolescence and bleeding	▶ Fish ▶ Meat ▶ Vegetables ▶ Whole grain products
Fluoride (F)	▶ Skeleton ▶ Hardening of tooth enamel ▶ Caries prevention	▶ Cooking and table salt with added fluoride
Iodine (J)	▶ Component of thyroid hormone ▶ Iodine deficiency during pregnancy ▶ Goitre due to iodine deficiency	▶ Saltwater fish ▶ Iodine salt
Zinc (Zn)	▶ Blood sugar regulation ▶ Anti-inflammatory ▶ Stabilization of cell walls ▶ Strengthening of immune system	▶ Meat ▶ Fish ▶ Shellfish ▶ Eggs ▶ Dairy products ▶ Offal

race Elements	Function	Food Sources
opper (Cu)	▶ Component of many enzymes ▶ Supports iron utilization and tissue growth	▶ Meat ▶ Fish ▶ Shellfish ▶ Fungi ▶ Beans ▶ Whole grain products ▶ Nuts
Manganese (Mn)	▶ Bone construction ▶ Construction of connective tissue ▶ Cholesterol formation ▶ Carbohydrate metabolism	▶ Whole grain products ▶ Soya beans ▶ Bananas
Selenium (Se)	▶ Antioxidant effect ▶ Counteracts poisonous substances, such as mercury ▶ Possibly prevents cancer	▶ Liver ▶ Flesh ▶ Offal ▶ Pulses ▶ Nuts
Chromium (Cr)	▶ Utilization of carbohydrates ▶ Regulation of blood sugar level	▶ Fruit ▶ Potatoes ▶ Whole grain products ▶ Vegetables ▶ Nuts

tegut

3.5 Fluid Balance

Water is an essential part of our diets. There are many reasons to drink several liters of water per day, whether just to maintain good health or to try to lose weight. Man can survive for weeks without solid food, but just a few days without fluids can be

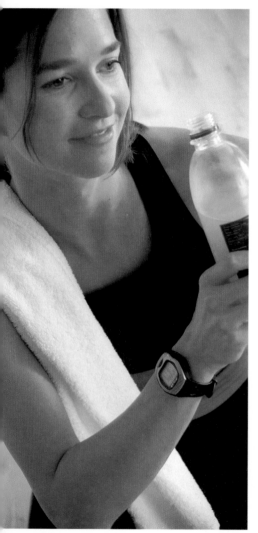

fatal. More than half of the body consists of water (about 38 – 47 liters) and it eliminates about 2.5l daily through sweat, urine, breathing and through the intestine.

An adequate fluid intake is essential to replace lost water. The more active a person is and the higher the ambient temperature, the more water the body needs.

Physical activity quickly raises the daily water requirement by a few liters, especially if carried out in hot conditions. Water has a fundamental, nutritional-physiological role. The most important reasons for an adequate water intake are listed below:

Table 11: Nine reasons to drink a lot of water

▶Water is an essential nutrient

▶Water makes one feel full

▶Water delivers nutrients to the cells

▶Water transports hormones and disease-fighting cells in the bloodstream

▶Water is necessary for many chemical reactions during digestion and metabolism

▶Water allows sweat production, which controls body temperature

▶Water protects tissues

▶Water lubricates joints

▶Water relieves constipation

3.6 Diets: No, thanks!

The term *diet* is a relatively general description for all special nutritional programs. It is used for both medically necessary diets and unnecessary or even unhealthy diets. There are diets that are only used for temporary weight loss and others that must be followed for life for health reasons. From a scientific point of view, diets are categorized as follows:

▶ Diets to prevent and manage certain diseases (e.g., diabetes)
▶ Diets for moral or ethical reasons (e.g., vegetarianism)
▶ Diets to lose weight

The latter is seen in a fat-burning context in advertising slogans (e.g., "Your dream figure in just four weeks," or "slimming – 4 kg in only one week"), which are completely untrue and ridiculous. Many people even put on more weight after a diet than they lost during it. Leading nutritional scientists even see weight-loss diets as the reason for obesity.

It is certainly possible to lose 3-4 kg in one week. This does not mean that body fat has been lost, though. In most cases, there is even a percentage increase in body fat, as on a crash diet when what is lost is water.

tegut

Furthermore, the body is not particularly healthy during and after a diet. Someone who works on his or her feet and who doesn't want to lose energy should only reduce weight on a long-term basis.

? Why can 3-4 kg not be lost in a Week?

To break down 1kg of body fat, about 7,000 calories must be eliminated on a low-fat and specific diet, or burned up in appropriate exercise. This still appears relatively realistic if one eats 1,000 kcal less than the body needs for a period of seven days.

A normal person requires between 1,800 and 2,800 kcal per day depending on age, height, gender, body weight and physical activity level. How can 3 or 4 kg of body fat be lost in one week?

For a fat reduction of 4 kg, 28,000 kcal must be eliminated. Even by fasting and doing extra exercise, it is impossible to cut out 4,000 calories per day. This sample calculation shows how unrealistic these popular crash diets are.

Yo-yo Effect

From a medical and health point of view, there are many disadvantages to crash dieting. Many people have already had the experience of weighing more after dieting than they did before. For a long time, nutritional scientists have argued that it is not possible to achieve lasting weight loss with short-term "crash" diets.

It is easy to explain a weight increase after coming off a diet from a physical point of view. The human body is always trying to maintain the same weight.

tegut

When little food is available, it starts to manage with less. That is why when on a diet, the body starts to run on the "back burner", i.e., the basal metabolic rate is lowered. After a certain time during the diet, the body starts to mobilize its reserves, which are not primarily body fat but those energy reserves that are the easiest to mobilize (e.g., proteins, glycogen from the liver and muscles).

The fat deposits are only mobilized by the body as the very last resort. As every gram of glycogen is attached to 4 g of water, the rapid weight loss at the start of a diet is only due to the loss of water. Once the glycogen reserves are burned away, the body begins to burn muscle protein and fat. A low-protein diet with very few calories accompanied by very little exercise leads mainly to rapid muscle breakdown.

When the weight loss goal has been reached, the body stays on the "back burner" for a while afterward. So, until it has gotten used to "normal service" again, the body receives far too much food, which it stores as fat, almost as reserves for hard times to come. This is why more weight is put on after a diet than was lost. The proportion of fat tissue has also greatly increased in most cases, as the diet has mainly broken down muscle. This mechanism is often called the "*yo-yo effect.*"

There are a whole series of other weight-loss measures besides dieting that should definitely be avoided, as in the long term they do not lead to successful results.

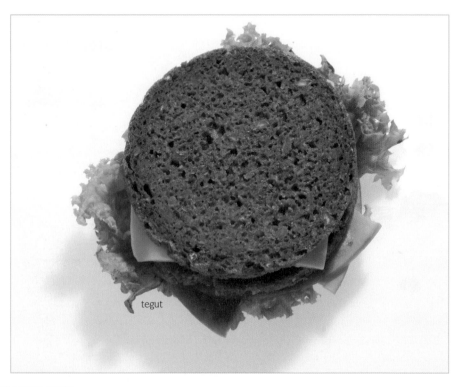

tegut

Table 12: Ineffective fat-burning methods

Slimming Food	▶ No taste ▶ No learning process as to how to deal with normal food ▶ Only short-term weight loss
Appetite suppressant/ removal methods	▶ Health risks (eating disorders, tachycardia, outbreaks of sweating) ▶ Weight loss due to lost water. Only short-term weight loss
Cigarettes	▶ Damaging side effects of nicotine ▶ Decreased oxygen uptake ▶ Diminished endurance ability
Eating half portions	▶ Under-satisfaction leads to low blood sugar level ▶ Starving at next meal-time ▶ Not enough food for optimal fat burning

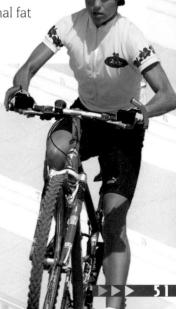

3.7 Nutrition Tips for Fat Burning

Your slimming goal should be realistic; it can be discouraging not to reach an over-ambitious target (a loss of 1kg every 2-3 weeks is realistic). Along with a balanced and qualitatively and quantitatively correct diet, sufficient exercise should also be taken. Furthermore, never go shopping on an empty stomach; if you are hungry, you always fill your trolley more than you should!

Table 13: Nutrition tips for fat burning

Nutrition Tips	Commentary
Keep an eating log	An eating log helps you to establish where the weaknesses in your diet are (i.e., too much sugar, too much fat, too much alcohol).
Change your eating habits	A change of eating habits means a qualitative change for many people. For some, it means a quantitative change, too, of course, i.e., eating less.
Drink abundantly	Drink at least 3 liters per day, if possible mineral water or unsweetened herbal and fruit teas. Avoid high-sugar lemonades and fruit juices. Alcoholic drinks also have a high calorie content.
Eat sensibly	Don't eat high-calorie snacks (e.g., crisps, peanuts, chocolates) out of boredom.

Nutrition Tips	Commentary
Avoid fatty food	Instead choose low-fat cheese, low-fat milk and low-fat sausage. Watch out for hidden fats in nuts, sausages and meats.
Snack on fruits and vegetables between meals	If you feel a little hungry between meals, fruits and vegetables are suitable as they are filling, provide important minerals and vitamins and have few calories.
Sweetener in moderation	If you can't give up sugar, you can replace it with sweeteners in moderation.
Eat slowly	You should always eat slowly. The brain only registers the first signals of saturation from the metabolism after 15-20 minutes.
Small meals	Eat five smaller meals a day instead of three large ones.
Avoid white flour and sugar	Instead, take in carbohydrates in the form of whole grain products, rice, pasta or potatoes.
A glass of water before eating	This will calm a raging appetite.

3.8 Nutrition and Endurance Training

If you participate in endurance activities, you should make sure that your energy and fluid intake is adequate.

Energy Balance – eating before and after Training

The body's glycogen and fat reserves are reduced in line with the duration of the endurance load. While at low intensity, the mobilization of the fat deposits takes place (adipolysis); at peak loading, the glycogen reserves are drawn upon. The ability to burn fat can be learned, incidentally. Good endurance athletes can quickly draw upon their fat reserves, thereby sparing the glycogen reserves.

Tips

Nutrition tips and endurance sport:

▶ A full stomach precludes abdominal respiration. The last meal should therefore be 2-3 hours before training.

▶ You shouldn't train on an empty stomach though, as efficiency is reduced due to a lowered carbohydrate uptake and a reduction of the blood sugar level.

▶ An endurance athlete's diet is largely made up of carbohydrates, i.e., of a lot of bread (with pasta, rice, pulses, vegetables and fruit). The nutrient ratio for endurance sports should be as follows: 60% carbohydrate, 15% protein, 25% fat. Under extreme conditions, many top sportspeople increase the carbohydrate percentage up to 80%.

▶ After every intensive endurance training session, the carbohydrate stores should be replenished quickly.

Fluid Balance

If you don't drink during exercise, the body falls back on water in the tissues and the blood. The muscles are then not adequately supplied with oxygen and nutrients, thus leading to dizziness, blood circulation disorders or muscle cramps.

Top sportspeople can lose more than 2 liters of fluid in one hour in intensive competition at high temperatures. That is why before, during and after training or competition sufficient fluid intake is vital. Under extreme conditions (high temperatures, sun, competition), athletes should drink 150-250 ml of fluid every 20-30 minutes.

If you do endurance training to burn fat, no additional fluid should be drunk during training that lasts less than 60 minutes and where the temperature is not too high. A fluid loss of 0.5 – 1.0 liters does not affect efficiency.

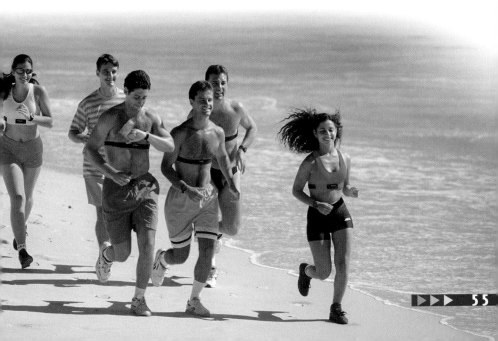

For long training sessions at high temperatures, additional fluid intake is advisable. Drinks that are too cold, too sugary and especially alcoholic should be avoided. Mineral water, fruit squashes (50:50 juice to water ratio) and drinks with a carbohydrate percentage of 8-12% have proved to be appropriate.

Electrolyte or isotonic drinks are controversial, on the other hand. It has been reported from the sport of beach volleyball that since the players have stopped drinking hypertonic and isotonic drinks, replacing them with mineral water combined with salt biscuits, they now suffer practically no cramping. This currently seems to be the simplest and cheapest way of preventing cramps caused by salt deficiency.

? What are isotonic Drinks?

Isotonic drinks are soft drinks which contain added minerals, water and sometimes vitamins, sugar, sweeteners or carbon dioxide. Isotonic drinks are especially popular among endurance athletes for replacing lost water and minerals.

Isotonic Drinks
Isotonic drinks possess the same osmosis level (particle concentration) as blood plasma. As the concentration corresponds to that of blood, during long endurance sessions (> 1 hour), the fluid is easily taken up by the body.

Hypotonic Drinks (hypo = less)
The particle concentration of hypotonic drinks is lower. Hypotonic drinks (e.g. tea, water, mineral water) possess a lower osmosis level than blood plasma, i.e., they are even more suitable for rapid fluid absorption than isotonic drinks.

Hypertonic Drinks (hyper = more)

Hypertonic drinks have a higher osmosis level than blood plasma, i.e., the particle concentration is higher. These drinks are more concentrated than the blood, they deprive the body of water and are therefore unsuitable for the sportsperson.

An endurance athlete who trains for 30-60 minutes in order to lose weight does not require special fitness or isotonic drinks. Mineral water or diluted apple juice are ideal for replacing the potassium and sodium lost by sweating. Incidentally, thirst means fluid deficiency. If you wait until you feel thirsty before drinking, it will be too late, as your efficiency will have already dropped.

Tip

Drinking correctly during endurance sport

▶ Drink slowly
▶ The drink should not be too cold
▶ No alcohol during sport. This removes water from the body.
▶ Avoid juices with additional sugar
▶ Choose a low carbon dioxide mineral water

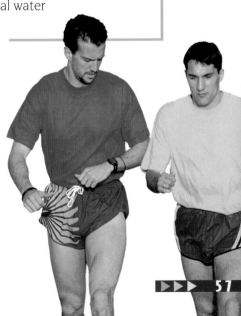

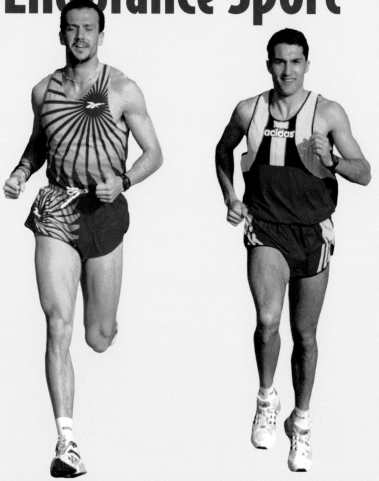

The Demands of Endurance Sport

The physical and psychosocial demands involved in endurance sport are firstly very individual and secondly not lasting. For example, the demands on the beginner in the conditioning, coordination and mental areas are very high in the first few training sessions. The exercise initially requires a lot of strength. Self-motivation and great perseverance are required not to give up immediately.

Objectively identical physical demands (e.g., 1,000 m swimming; 50 minutes cycling) are definitely perceived differently just a few weeks later. As a result of the first training effects, training will soon start to seem much easier.

However, there are some typical general endurance sport demands in the areas of conditioning, coordination and mental, which will be described below:

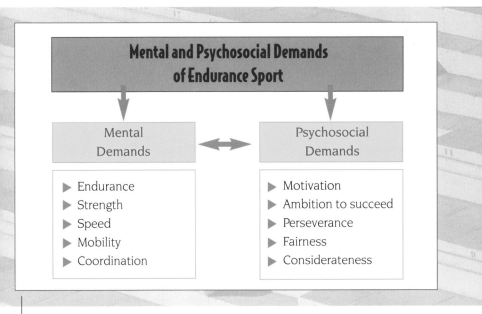

Figure 3: Mental and psychosocial demands of endurance sport

4.1 Physical Demands

There is no general conditioning or coordination profile for endurance athletes, as there are quite clear differences between endurance sports in terms of main conditioning demands and coordination.

This is firstly due to the various surfaces or media, on or in which the sport is carried out: e.g., snow (cross-country skiing), water (swimming, water jogging), concrete (inline skating) or forest trails (running).

Secondly, it can be a result of the different conditioning and coordination demands of each sport. While running, hiking and inline skating mainly develop the strength endurance of the leg muscles; swimming and cross-country skiing are whole-body sports, as they also train the arms and torso.

The general conditioning in endurance sport comprises the main demand forms of endurance, strength, speed and mobility. As expected, endurance is the most important of these, and the proficiency level of the above four conditioning abilities are also greatly influenced by that of coordination.

The three basic physical principles of endurance, strength and speed should not be considered in isolation for each individual endurance sport. Of the resulting combinations – strength-endurance, speed-endurance and speed-strength – strength endurance plays the most important role in endurance sport, as the speed component is negligible.

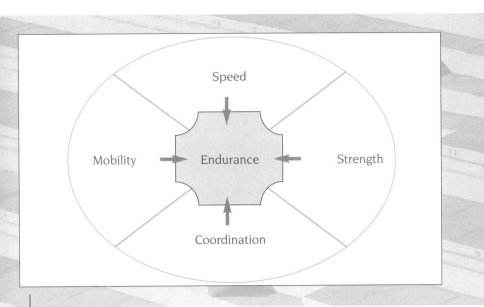

Figure 4: Conditioning and coordination demands in endurance sport

There is a special, endurance-sport-specific conditioning, plus sport-specific coordination demands (e.g., reaction and balance in inline skating and cross-country skiing), and as good as possible mobility, particularly in the knees, hips and, in some sports, also the shoulder area (e.g., swimming).

This special conditioning ability of a well-trained endurance athlete can be described as follows:

- ▶ Good general aerobic endurance
- ▶ Well-developed strength endurance, particularly in the leg muscles
- ▶ Good mobility in the knee and hip joints
- ▶ Well-developed coordination abilities relevant to the endurance sport concerned

The individual conditioning and coordination demand forms are briefly examined below. In the next chapter, the main conditioning endurance forms are dealt with separately and thoroughly, according to their importance (cf. chapter 5).

4.1.1 Strength

Strength as a physical value is defined as the product of mass times acceleration ($F = m \times a$). From a physiological point of view, a difference should be made between static and dynamic strength. *Static* strength refers to the muscle tension that can be employed deliberately against a resistance in a given position – without the origin and insertion of the muscle moving toward each other.

Dynamic strength is defined by the mass that can be moved during a motion sequence. Both forms of strength are based on the interaction of the central nervous system (CNS) and the skeletal musculature.

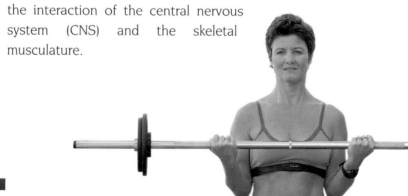

Dynamic muscle strength is the crucial form for endurance sports. Out of the three types of strength – *maximal strength, speed strength and strength endurance* – strength endurance is the most important for endurance sport. Speed strength, or the ability to overcome resistance as fast as possible, is not relevant to endurance exercise for fat burning. Strength endurance, on the other hand, is performance-critical, particularly for long endurance workouts.

The lack of strength endurance in the lower limbs is the greatest performance limiting factor for many endurance athletes, e.g., in mountain biking or running, resulting in premature tiredness. Strength endurance in the torso and arm muscles is also extremely important in swimming and cross-country skiing.

Regular strength endurance training brings many advantages for competitive endurance athletes. For the fitness-oriented recreational athlete who just wants to lose weight, endurance training in itself soon leads to an improvement in strength endurance, so that additional strength training may not actually be necessary. In particular, training with increasing and decreasing intensities (cycling, spinning, running), technique (water jogging) or the combination of up and downhill (cycling, in-line skating) leads to an improvement of strength endurance in the lower limbs in themselves.

Sand is an ideal training surface for developing the strength and strength endurance components for runners and walkers. In every training session, the relevant basic abilities are improved, running on sand always presents increased resistance and considerably more strength than that required on the road or in the gym. Regular training on sand brings relatively rapid adaptation of the foot, calf and thigh muscles, so that initial symptoms of fatigue soon decrease noticeably after regular workouts. Here is a short overview of the special benefits of training on sand:

Table 14: Benefits of endurance training on sand

- ► Doing bare-foot sports strengthens the often neglected foot muscles

- ► Exercising on sand is a kind of rehabilitation from an orthopedic point of view

- ► The constantly changing surface underfoot develops the coordination ability in particular

- ► Exercise on sand strengthens very effectively and particularly improves the strength endurance of the lower limbs

- ► Increased muscle building and a softer, cushioned surface leads to fewer injuries

- ► Peak loading of the ankles is reduced due to a longer contact time with the ground

- ► The lower limb joints – ankle, knee and hip joints – receive less stress compared to indoor sport

- ► The constantly changing surface strengthens the muscles of the lower extremities and torso; malpositions can be compensated for in this way

- ► High cardiovascular loading can lead to an increase in the aerobic/anaerobic threshold

- ► Injured athletes can continue to train to some degree due to the therapeutic effect of the sand

4.1.2 Speed

The physical definition of *speed* is distance per unit of time. Physiologically, speed is the ability to carry out movements – appropriate mobility, nervous system and skeletal musculature processes – as fast as possible under certain given conditions. Compared to endurance and strength, speed plays a relatively unimportant role in endurance exercise.

4.1.3 Mobility

The term mobility is usually used to refer to joint mobility. This can be understood as the arbitrary possible range of movement of a joint. Mobility is often equated with such terms as *flexibility*, *mobility, suppleness* or *stretchability*.

Mobility is a combination of the stretchability of muscles, joint capsules and tendons, and the suppleness, or the structure and function, of the bony joints. A high degree of mobility first requires high amplitude in the joint concerned, which results in an extension of the acceleration distance.

This enables various movements to be carried out more accurately and, above all, more economically. Secondly, good mobility prevents injury. The danger of muscle, bone, ligament and joint capsule injury is reduced by well-developed mobility.

Good mobility even makes learning new sport-specific movements, e.g., swimming techniques, inline skating or cross-country skiing, easier. Mobility training in the cool-down phase also lowers the heightened muscle tone and brings general physical relaxation.

4.1.4 Coordination

Coordination or *agility* is defined as the co-action of the Central Nervous System (CNS) and the skeletal muscles within a certain movement sequence. There are seven coordination abilities: differentiation, interoperability, reaction speed, spatial orientation, jumping, balance and rhythm abilities.

Only good coordination allows complex movement tasks to be tackled successfully, i.e., correctly and precisely. The coordination demands of various endurance sports are completely different, however, depending on the complexity of the movement (e.g., arm and leg technique for swimming) and depending on the surface underfoot (e.g., snow, forest trails).

4.2 Psychosocial Demands

The psychosocial demands of endurance sport should not be underestimated. It depends entirely on the individual whether they enjoy exercise or not. This is, though, the pre-requisite for a regular and long-term exercise program.

The level of motivation has a great effect on the psychomotor execution of sporting movement; first indirectly on the conditioning level and second, directly on the athlete's mental qualities, such as motivation, ambition, concentration or the handling of success and failure. If the sport is not carried out alone but in pairs or a larger group, there are also social demands on the endurance athlete.

To sum up, the psychosocial demands of endurance sport, particularly in the initial training sessions seem fairly high for several reasons:

- ▶ Overcoming one's weaker self
- ▶ New movement experiences
- ▶ Learning new techniques
- ▶ Living up to one's own expectations
- ▶ Willingness to perform
- ▶ Adjustment to training partner
- ▶ Consideration and fairness

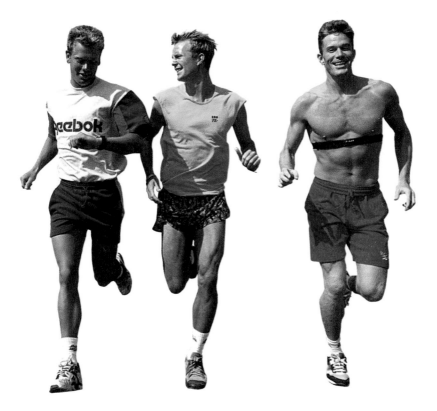

Endurance Training

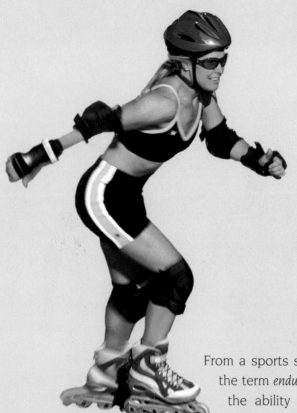

From a sports science point of view, the term *endurance* is used to mean the ability to maintain a given physical load without serious signs of tiredness for as long as possible. This ability is also called the ability to resist fatigue. The main demand form of endurance is also assigned to subsequent rapid regeneration or recovery ability.

endurance = ability to resist fatigue + recovery ability

5.1 Forms of Endurance

From a training science point of view, endurance is subdivided according to various criteria. We differentiate between:

▶ The size of the participating muscle-mass (general-local)
▶ Type of energy supply (aerobic-anaerobic)
▶ Function of the skeletal muscles (dynamic-static)
▶ Duration of the load (short, medium, long)

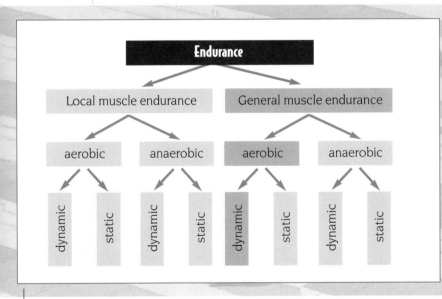

Figure 5: Diagram of the different endurance forms

General endurance means the ability to resist fatigue when large muscle groups are used – more than a sixth to a seventh of the whole skeletal musculature – during whole body movement (e.g., lower limb musculature when running).

Local endurance refers to very small muscle groups of less than a sixth to a seventh of the entire skeletal musculature. For fat burning, it is important to address as large a muscle group as possible, in order to burn as much energy as possible, for instance, general muscle endurance is important here.

The type of energy supply determines whether the endurance form is aerobic or aerobic. In *aerobic* (aerobic = oxygen dependent) *endurance*, enough oxygen is available to the musculature to burn glycogen for the work to be performed. If the glycogen reserves are used up after longer loads (over 30 minutes), the necessary energy is provided by the breakdown of fats using oxygen.

In *anaerobic* (anaerobic = without oxygen) *endurance*, the energy required for muscle work is supplied in spite of a high oxygen debt, where lactic acid is formed during the anaerobic glycolysis of sugar. Under long, intensive loads, this leads to the acidaemia of the muscles with concomitant lactate formation (lactate = lactic acid salt). During fat burning, the aim should be to engage the largest possible muscle mass for as long as possible in order to burn as much energy as possible.

Lactate, aerobic and anaerobic threshold

Under physical loading, the body produces lactate. This waste product is not formed by the skeletal muscles, but by the heart, kidneys and liver. Up to a certain loading intensity, the body breaks down lactate faster than it forms it. The point at which the lactate formed by the body can no longer be broken down is called the *anaerobic threshold*. Once this has been crossed, the lactate produced by the body can not be broken down fast enough and the blood lactate values rise sharply. A prolonged lactic acid buildup leads to the acidification of the muscle, which inhibits several biological reactions within the muscle, resulting in abandonment or reduction of the too-high loading intensity.

Approximate values for the lactate concentration in the blood (mmol/l)

< 2 mmol/l:	aerobic training load
2 mmol/l:	aerobic threshold
> 4 mmol/l:	anaerobic threshold
> 2 mmol/l:	anaerobic training load

The area between the aerobic threshold and the anaerobic threshold is also termed the *aerobic/anaerobic transition* area. This is where lactate production and removal are held in balance.

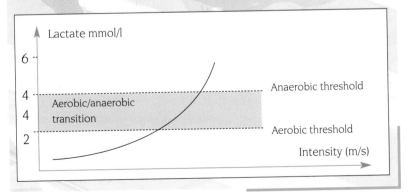

According to the type of load (stationary or moving), endurance can also be *static* or *dynamic*. This has an important influence on the energy supply. While in static training, the blood and, therefore, the oxygen supply to the muscles slows down (increasingly anaerobic energy supply), during dynamic work the blood supply is assured for longer. Dynamic endurance training is appropriate for losing weight.

Endurance training is further sub-divided into *short*, *middle* and *long duration*. This in turn has a decisive influence on the energy supply. Short-term endurance is the ability to resist fatigue during sporting effort lasting between 45 seconds and 2 minutes, where energy is supplied anaerobically. Medium duration covers effort lasting between 2 and 8 minutes, where anaerobic and aerobic supplies are more or less balanced. Long-duration endurance covers efforts lasting more than 8 minutes, where the energy supply is almost completely aerobic. Long-duration endurance is the most suitable for fat burning. The table below shows the percentages of aerobic and anaerobic energy supplies for various athletics running events. Variations are possible, especially in the middle distance events, according to the fitness of the individual and the loading intensity.

	100 m	200 m	400 m	800 m	1.000 m	1.500 m	5.000 m	10.000 m	Marathon
Aerobic	5 %	10 %	25 %	45 %	50 %	65 %	90 %	95 %	99 %
Anaerobic	95 %	90 %	75 %	55 %	50 %	35 %	10 %	5 %	1 %

Figure 6: Percentages of aerobic and anaerobic energy supplies using athletic running events

Endurance training for weight loss is mainly general, aerobic, dynamic and long-duration

5.2 Energy Supply

To reduce weight through exercise (muscle activity), a "fuel" is required, whose splitting enables muscles to contract (muscle shortening and/or muscle tensing). This fuel is called ATP (Adenosine TriPhosphate). This is an energy-rich phosphate compound that liberates energy when split.

However, the amount of ATP stored in the muscle cells is extremely small, so, as the muscles can only be fuelled by ATP, the other energy reserves (carbohydrate, protein, fat) must also ultimately supply ATP. Fat is the largest of these energy reserves and supplies the energy during long loads.

If we consider the intensity and duration of the load, it is clear that the phosphate compounds supply energy very fast (< 10 seconds) under very high loads. Carbohydrates provide relatively large amounts of energy under sub-maximal and medium loads of short to medium duration (10 seconds – 8 minutes). Fats are the best energy providers for long-lasting, lowintensity loads.

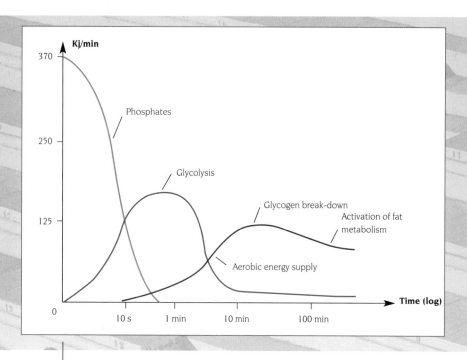

Figure 7: Energy supply forms at maximal demand according to time

The three energy sources can be divided into aerobic (with oxygen) and anaerobic (without oxygen) supplies, and also lactic (with the build-up of lactate in the muscle cells) and alactic (without lactate production) energy supply.

There are four time phases, each dominated by one of the energy supply forms:

► The burning of the phosphate compounds plays a decisive role in the first 10 seconds. Energy is supplied without oxygen and without the accumulation of lactate (anaerobic-alactic energy supply).

► Between 30 seconds and 2 minutes, the burning of carbohydrates (glycolysis) dominates, mainly without oxygen and with the buildup of lactate (anaerobic-lactic energy supply). The more intensive the training, the faster the glycogen reserves are emptied, the sooner fatigue sets in and more oxygen is required, resulting in more rapid breathing.

► From 2-8 minutes, aerobic glycogen utilization dominates. The energy supply takes place with oxygen and without lactate buildup (aerobic-alactic energy supply).

► The fourth form of energy supply is the burning of fat. Depending to the fitness of the individual, this initially takes place after around 45 minutes with oxygen and without lactate buildup (aerobic-alactic energy supply).

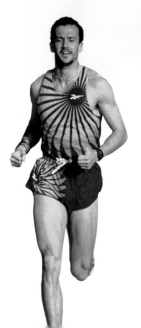
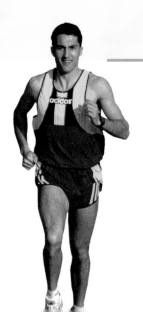

Table 15: An overview of the energy reserves of the human body (phosphate compounds, carbohydrates and fats)

	Energy Reserves in kcal (30-yr-old man; 75kg)	Load intensity	Duration of energy supply	Energy supply
Phosphate bonds (ATP)	About 5 kcal	Maximal	< 10 s	Anaerobic-alactic
Carbohydrates (glycolysis)	About 1.200 kcal	Sub-maximal	45 s-2 min	Anaerobic-lactic
Carbohydrates (glykogen break-down)		Average	2-8 min	Aerobic-alactic
Fat	About 50.000 kcal	Low	> 45 min	Aerobic-alactic

Steady State

Fat burning requires a loading intensity that guarantees an aerobic energy supply. This is the only way that oxygen uptake and oxygen consumption are in balance, or a steady state. In apparent *steady state*, as the name suggests, the balance is not real. Oxygen uptake is a little higher than the amount of oxygen provided, resulting in a slight oxygen debt.

5.3 Heart Rate Zones

Training can take place in several different heart rate zones. The categories and terms are not always consistent.

Five zones are usually given, each with its own percentage range.

Table 16: Heart rate zones

Number	Name	Maximal Heart Rate (MHR)	Training emphasis
Zone 1	Health zone	50-60 %	▶ Ideal for beginners ▶ Stabilization of the cardiovascular system
Zone 2	Fat burning zone	60-70 %	▶ Improvement of the cardiovascular system ▶ The body consumes more fat than carbohydrates
Zone 3	Aerobic zone	70-80 %	▶ Improvement of breathing and circulation ▶ Optimal for increasing endurance (aerobic training) ▶ More carbohydrates than fats burned
Zone 4	Anaerobic threshold zone	80-90 %	▶ Training for competitive athletes ▶ Oxygen demand can no longer be met (anaerobic training) ▶ Upward shift of the anaerobic threshold
Zone 5	Red Zone	90-100 %	▶ Only for elite athletes ▶ Very dangerous for recreational athletes (heart)

Most beginners and all inexperienced recreational athletes initially choose a load that is too high. This means that performances do not improve over the long term and overloading, or even injuries, can result. If you want to lose weight and burn fat through endurance exercise, you should train mostly in the fat-burning zone (60-70% of maximal heart rate).

As soon as you start to train and remain in the aerobic zone, as a percentage, more carbohydrates are burned than fats. If you train regularly and persistently in the fat-burning zone while following a low-fat diet, the body is forced to turn to its (fat) reserves.

5.4 Training Methods

Endurance training means training without stopping over a period of 20-35 minutes. There are a whole series of endurance training methods:

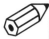

- ▶   Continuity method
- ▶   Extensive interval method
- ▶   Intensive interval method
- ▶   Fartlek
- ▶   Repetition method

If you are doing endurance sport with the aim of burning fat, the most important methods for you are the *extensive interval training* and *continuity methods*, as well as low to average intensity Fartlek training.

Endurance training loading intensity

Loading Duration (Stimulus Duration)
Given in seconds, minutes or hours (e.g., 40 mins running).

Loading Volume (Training Volume)
Total amount of loading stimuli in one training session or over a long training period (micro and macro cycle) (e.g., three hours/weeks).

Loading Intensity (Training Intensity)
The strength of an individual loading stimulus. For endurance sport, the intensity is given either by speed, heart rate or the blood lactate value. Beginners usually start training at too high an intensity. This is unwise if weight loss is desired, as the body gets tired too quickly. Further negative consequences of a too-high training intensity are: muscle stiffness, prolonged recovery time and, in many cases, an increased risk of infection.

Loading Density (Stimulus Density)
Time gap between the individual loading stimuli. Expressed as the rest period between the loading stimuli.

Training Frequency
Number of training units in a training period (e.g., 4 x/week).

Continuity Method

The *continuity method* is a consistent load without rest over a long period of time. The training should last at least 30 minutes, except for beginners. The loading intensity should be between 60 and 80% of the maximal performance ability (VO_2 max).

The continuous method mainly trains the metabolism, particularly the fat metabolism. In addition, the blood circulation (capillarisation) of the loaded muscles is improved on a long-term basis.

Interval Method

The *interval method* is generally understood to mean training with loading breaks, i.e., the load is not continuous, but broken up with frequent rest periods (intervalbreakss). The rest periods between the intervals should be long enough to recover well, but the pulse should not drop too far. This is known as the "beneficial rest". The rests should be active, i.e., there should be a light load, such as gentle running, cycling, swimming or aqua jogging.

As an approximation, the pulse rate should only drop to between 120 – 140 beats/min. A set is made up of a certain number of repetitions. After each *set,* there is a longer break than between the individual repetitions. We distinguish between *extensive* and *intensive interval training,* according to the intensity at which the interval training is carried out.

Extensive interval training is carried out at an intensity of 60-80% of maximal loading. The duration of the intervals is about 4-8 minutes and the number of repetitions is 10-20. Extensive interval training develops both the cardiovascular system and the metabolism to a high level. This training is most suitable for beginners to increase the load duration in a given sport.

Intensive interval training is carried out at a high intensity, between 80 and 95% of maximal loading, and in the *repetition method* (long rests until nearly complete recovery) even with a loading intensity of 90-100%.

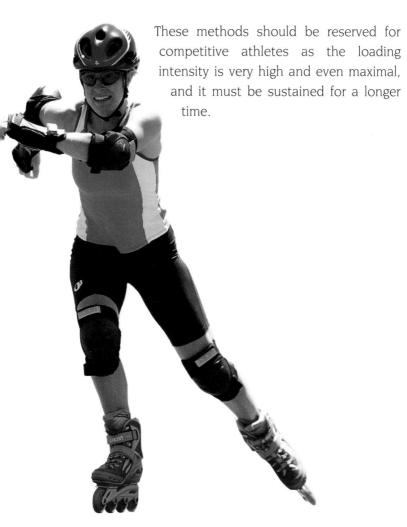

These methods should be reserved for competitive athletes as the loading intensity is very high and even maximal, and it must be sustained for a longer time.

Fartlek

In Fartlek training, the loading intensity is changed at irregular intervals, they can range from quite short to maximal. The loading change can be altered according to individual fitness or external conditions (e.g., hills). Recovery is active.

As it is actually a continuous load of constantly changing levels, Fartlek is a type of endurance training method and is treated as such in coaching literature.

Fartlek is eminently suitable for building up complex endurance performance ability, i.e., both in adaptations in the cardiovascular system and in the metabolism and muscular energy supplies.

Conclusion

Endurance training for fat burning should be carried out at least three times per week in order to boost the active metabolic rate and the calorie requirement, as well as to maintain and improve endurance performance ability. Above all, this requires long-duration and low-intensity training.

The endurance method at a load of 60-70% is the method of choice. The loading period should be at least 30-40 minutes. The extensive interval method can also be used, particularly at the start of the training process.

For the more advanced, Fartlek carried out at relatively low to average loading intensities is a motivating alternative. For recreational athletes, there is a danger of overloading with the other methods.

Muscle Soreness

There are 400 skeletal muscles in the human body, whose movement is carried out over the tendons on bones and joints. Muscles can support enormous loads, as long as they are regularly loaded and trained. This is why novice and returning athletes often complain of muscle soreness, usually 1 or 2 days after the first training sessions.

Muscle soreness is a clear sign of overloading and overexertion. Muscle soreness is not caused, as was previously thought, by lactate, but rather by micro-injuries to the muscles due to excessive loading. Preventive measures against muscle soreness are:

▶ Warm-up
▶ Stretching and gentle running or swimming after the training session.
▶ Regular exercise
▶ Do not place untrained muscles under inordinately heavy or long loads
▶ Increase intensity and volume gradually
▶ Rub in circulation-promoting muscle oils before training

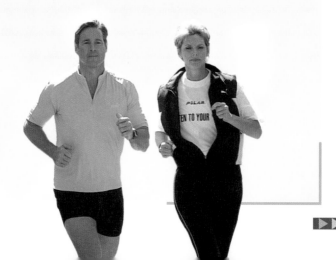

5.5 Load Monitoring

There are also several ways to monitor loading. In recreational sport, measuring the pulse rate and the subjective loading sensation are important.

The optimal Training Pulse Rate

There is a range of different formulae for calculating the optimal training pulse rate for each training form. Blanket pulse rate formulae have the disadvantage that they do not take into account individual pulse rates, so such formulae only give a rough guide.

That means that none of the pulse rate formulae available in sports science literature can be completely accurate in terms of individual conditions (age, training condition, resting pulse rate, maximal pulse rate, daily form).

▶ Heart rate = 180 – age
(Baum & Hollmann-Formula)
▶ Heart rate = 170 – 1/2 age ± 10 beats per minute
(Schmith & Israel formula)

More complex formulae, such as the Karvonen formula or the Lagerstrom & Graf formula, also include in their calculation the age-dependent maximal heart rate and the individual, training-conditioned resting pulse rate. Both produce similar results.

The Lagerstrom & Graf formula is:

Loading pulse rate = resting pulse rate +
[maximal pulse – age – resting pulse rate) x intensity%]

The maximal pulse rate should, if possible, be established or ascertained in a prior loading test.

If this is not the case, a rough approximation of the maximal pulse rate can be calculated according to the following formula:

Maximal pulse rate = 220 – age for men
Maximal pulse rate = 226 – age for women

The resting pulse rate (heart rate at absolute rest) is best measured in bed in the morning before getting up, as a few minutes after getting up, the pulse rate will already have gone up.

Training Pulse Rate for Fat Burning according to the Lagerstrom & Graf Formula

To reduce body fat, it is best to train in the fat-burning zone (60-70% of maximal heart rate). According to the Lagerstrom & Graf formula, the optimal pulse rate can be calculated as follows:

A 36-year-old woman has a resting pulse rate of 70 beats/min. Her calculated maximal pulse rate (226-age = maximal pulse) is 190 beats/min. From this maximal pulse rate, she subtracts her resting pulse rate of 70 beats/min and obtains a value of 120 beats/min. This value is then multiplied by 60 (lower limit of the fat-burning zone) and 70% (upper limit of the fat-burning zone) and added once more to the resting pulse rate.

Example 1: (36-yr-old female recreational athlete)	**Example 2:** (60-yr-old recreational athlete)
226 – 36 = 190 (maximal heart rate)	220 – 60 = 160 (maximal heart rate)
190 – 70 (resting pulse rate) = 120	160 – 80 (resting pulse rate) = 80
120 x 60 (%) = 72	80 x 60 (%) = 48
120 x 70 (%) = 84	80 x 70 (%) = 56
70 (resting pulse rate) + 72 = 142	80 (resting pulse rate) + 48 = 128
70 (resting pulse rate) + 84 = 154	80 (resting pulse rate) + 56 = 136
The recommended training pulse rate is therefore between **142 – 154 beats/min.**	The recommended training pulse rate is therefore between **128 – 136 beats/min**

There are easy-to-use pulse rate monitors available on the market (cf. Chapter 8) for on-going pulse rate monitoring. When taking the pulse rate without equipment, be aware that measuring by hand underestimates the real loading pulse rate, which is up to 10 beats/minute higher, particularly when measured after and not during the load.

If you still want to measure your own heart rate by pressing the carotid artery (carotid pulse rate) or the wrist (radialis pulse rate), you should do it directly after loading and always for the same duration (10 seconds), as otherwise these measurements are not comparable.

Subjective Loading Sensations

Another way of monitoring loading is subjective load evaluation using certain descriptions on given scales. The use of such scales calls for a high degree of physical awareness, though. A "verification" of the subjective loading sensation by measuring pulse rate is definitely necessary.

This kind of load monitoring depends on how you feel on the day, so there is a danger of overloading on days when one feels particularly fit. In general, according to duration, loading should be perceived as from "light to average" to "average to difficult," corresponding to values between "3" and "5" on a seven-step scale:

1 = very easy	5 = average to difficult
2 = easy	6 = difficult
3 = easy to average	7 = very difficult
4 = average	

The best Endurance Sports for Fat Burning

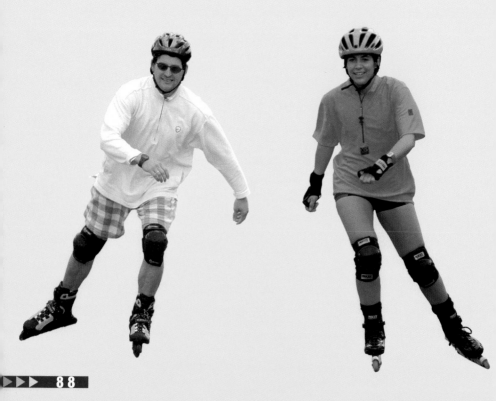

Endurance exercise is definitely the best form of physical activity for burning fat. But the calorie consumption of exercise should not be valued too highly. After playing badminton for one hour, a person weighing 70kg burns about 420 kcal and after one hour of easy swimming, 540 kcal. The same person uses up about 570 kcal from one hour of easy jogging (1km/7 mins) and from one hour of intensive jogging (1km/5 mins), about 840 kcal.

However, this compares to, for example, 150 g cream yogurt (about 185 kcal), a glass of beer (0.5 l, about 210 kcal) or 100 g milk chocolate (about 500 kcal). These examples show how quickly the burned calories can be replaced.

The energy balance actually turns out to be rather more advantageous, though, as the metabolic basal rate remains higher for a few hours after intense physical activity ("afterburner effect").

The examples given show once again that the combination of a low calorie diet with an appropriate endurance training program forms the basis of a successful fat-burning program.

Incidentally, if you don't lose any weight during the first weeks of training, and maybe even put on a little weight, don't be surprised. The cause is simply that muscle mass is heavier than fat. The weight gain just shows that muscles have been built up during training.

6.1 Choosing the right Endurance Sport

There is a whole range of very different sports. Alongside the classic sports of running, swimming, cycling and cross-country skiing, new sports, such as aqua jogging, inline skating, Spinning® and walking, have sprung up.

Furthermore, there are various fitness activities, such as aerobics, step or treadmill running, that are highly suitable alternative fat reduction methods. The answer to the question of the best alternative cannot and should not be the same for everyone. It is inter- and intra-individual.

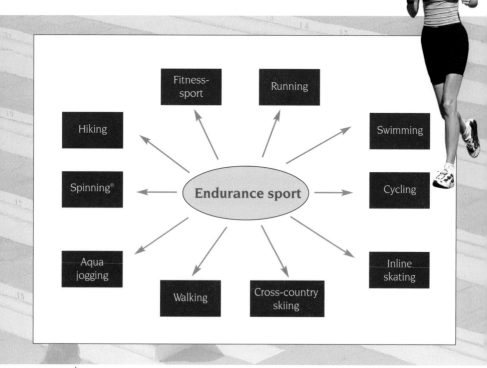

Figure 8: The best endurance sports for fat burning

Inter-individual means that the right endurance sport can turn out to be completely different from one person to another. So, for some, cycling or inline skating may be the ideal choice, while others may prefer running or, in winter, cross-country skiing.

Some may also favor the medium of water and enjoy swimming, aqua fitness or aqua jogging, while others are more at home in the fresh air, where they enjoy cycling or inline skating. Others yet may prefer a group training environment, e.g., aerobics, Spinning® and indoor cycling or they may seek an almost meditative peace and solitude in running or hiking.

Intra-individual differences in the choice of endurance sport are up to the individual. While one person may choose a low-impact endurance activity, such as aqua jogging or inline skating at the start of their weight reduction program, later on, the same person may prefer skiing or cross-country skiing on a winter sports holiday. Or, at another time, they may want to do sport to make contacts (socializing motive) and meet new people, and choose a group activity such as Spinning® or aerobics.

Choosing the right endurance activity is not easy for many people. There are many possibilities, depending on interests and motivation. Place of residence, organizational costs and seasons are also important considerations.

The current season will determine the choice of sport, i.e., cross-country skiing will only be possible in the winter months of December to March in most areas.

However, inline skating, mountain biking, cycling and hiking are the classic popular outdoor sports for the months of April to October. Practicing different sports throughout the year is advisable and possible. Indoor sports do not depend on the weather though, and Spinning®, swimming, aqua jogging, aqua fitness, aerobics and strength training can be carried out year-round.

Organizational costs also affect the choice of endurance activity. Buying equipment, such as a complete cross-country skiing outfit, should be well thought-out in advance. The venue where a sport will be carried out is also an important factor in decision-making.

Long journey times are demotivating in the long term. It is important that you should have as much fun as possible, because only if you are motivated to do a particular sport will you keep it up long term.

6.2 Running

Running is the original movement pattern and still the most popular endurance sport. According to various surveys, several million people jog twice a week or more.

As the optimal cardiovascular and fat-burning training form, running possesses some very specific advantages that explain its unique popularity:

- ▶ High calorie consumption
- ▶ Independence from sports clubs and facilities
- ▶ Running is possible almost anytime and anywhere, i.e., you can do it when you want from your own home
- ▶ Running brings rapid feelings of achievement
- ▶ Running is cheap (just the price of shoes and running clothes)
- ▶ Running is technically easy and quick to learn
- ▶ Running is possible at any age

Running for the Overweight

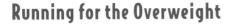

Running is not to be recommended unreservedly for the ever-growing number of people with weight or obesity problems, as it can lead to the overloading of the muscle-supporting bones, muscles, ligaments and tendons. The negative-dynamic muscle work on foot strike soon leads to overloading with well-known consequences (muscle soreness, joint pain, inactivity).

As the adaptation processes in the musculoskeletal system are substantially slower than those of the cardiovascular system, an improvement in endurance ability should not automatically imply a greater resilience of the tendons, ligaments and joints.

That is why the above population groups should go for other, more low-impact activities. Running should be started only when relevant adaptation processes in the muscle support system have taken place and/or after a suitable loss of weight.

The various alternative exercise forms also form the basis of and the introduction to a potential running career. After an introduction to the sport, the enjoyable alternative sports do not have to be abandoned, but may be continued alongside running training once or twice a week. After some time, the general physical condition may have improved so much from running and other sports that the running training intensity and volume can almost be increased without noticing.

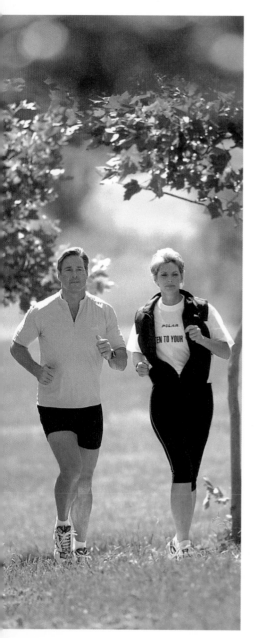

Two or three running sessions a week and one alternative sport session will further improve general aerobic basic endurance, reduce weight loss and form the basis for a long-lasting running career.

The right Shoes

The running shoe is, of course, the most important item of the running kit. It is not so easy to find a shoe that fits. Good advice from a specialist shop is recommended, preferably where a running-style analysis on a treadmill can be carried out.

Table 17: Tips for buying running shoes

▶ The way your used running or training shoes are worn down gives an experienced sales assistant important information about your individual running style

▶ It is best to buy shoes in the afternoon, as the foot swells up during the day

▶ Film a test run on the treadmill with a video camera

▶ It is better for the shoes to be too big than too small, as running makes the feet swell up quite a bit. There should be a finger's width between the big toe and the end of the shoe

▶ Very few people have two identically-sized feet. The largest one should be taken as standard

▶ If you wear orthotics in your running shoes, make sure the manufacturer's own insoles are removable, otherwise your feet will be too high in the shoe (danger of twisting your ankle)

▶ If you run regularly, you should possess at least one other pair to prevent injury

▶ Avoid breaking in new shoes in over-long training runs on over-hard surfaces

▶ Buy new shoes at least every 2,000 km

Technique

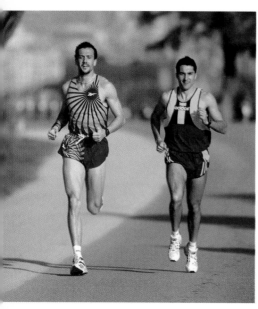

Running is not technically difficult in principle. However, many mistakes are made. While children have a naturally correct running style, many adults have unlearned the rhythm of running; many beginners are tensed up and overstride, which wastes power and energy.

The perfect running style is light, fluent and elegant. Only very few people run perfectly though. Many have their own individual style, due to their physique and muscular structure. A running style that is economical and as efficient as possible has the following features:

▶ Fluent and without overstriding

▶ Erect and slightly forward-inclined upper body

▶ Hips are tilted slightly forward

▶ Head is slightly raised and looking ahead

▶ Shoulders are loose, relaxed and still
(no swinging movement)

▶ Elbows are at a right-angles

▶ Hands are loose

Everyone can improve their running style. A second pair of eyes in the shape of a training partner, a sports teacher or athletics coach or a video running style analysis during a running seminar can be helpful.

Training

Beginning runners should run slowly in the first few weeks, for too much too soon brings no advantage, rather the opposite. Always remember the following training tips:

- ▶ Wear good running shoes and functional training clothes
- ▶ Warm up (fast walking and loose jogging and stretching) before every training session
- ▶ Start training on a flat surface
- ▶ To start with, run deliberately slowly
- ▶ The training method is: extensive intervals of running and walking recovery
- ▶ Monitor the duration of the running and walking recovery
- ▶ Without suitable recovery, training progress is not possible
- ▶ At least one rest day between training sessions
- ▶ Breathe as naturally as possible through the nose and mouth
- ▶ No large meals two hours before training
- ▶ Cool-down (gentle walking or jogging and stretching) after every training session

Below is a rough running training plan for an untrained beginner. The aim is to be able to run for 30 minutes after 10 weeks. Depending on individual fitness condition, you may start at the second or third week, or even skip a week in the case of rapid progress.

You don't have to stick strictly to the plan. Training should take place three times a week with a rest day in between. There is a 11/2 minute walking recovery period between the two intervals.

1. Week	6 x 2 min	running
2. Week	6 x 3 min	running
3. Week	6 x 4 min	running
4. Week	4 x 6 min	running
5 Week	4 x 8 min	running
6. Week	3 x 10 min	running
7. Week	3 x 10 min	running
8. Week	2 x 15 min	running
9. Week	1 x 20 min	running
	1 x 10 min	running
10. Week	30 min	running

Typical running injuries and problems are muscle cramps, inflammation of the sole of the foot, shin splints, Achilles tendon tears, adductor pulls, blisters, pulled ligaments, sciatic pain, mid-foot pain.

The above injuries and problems are quite easy to avoid and are mostly caused by:

- ▶ Too rapid an increase in training volume
- ▶ Too much training (over-training)
- ▶ No stretching or strengthening of the participating muscle groups
- ▶ No warm-up or cool-down
- ▶ Incorrect running style
- ▶ Badly-fitting footwear

6.3 Swimming

Swimming is healthy, weight-reducing and recreational at the same time. It is a whole-body exercise that provides endurance and strength-endurance training for many muscle groups. The most important advantage, especially for the overweight who want to lose weight by swimming are:

- ▶ It is a whole-body exercise that trains nearly all important muscle groups
- ▶ It is a life-long sport that can be continued into very old age
- ▶ Low injury risk
- ▶ As it is low-impact, it is ideally suited for the overweight or those with joint problems, as when swimming, you don't have to support your own body weight; there is no loading on joints and bones
- ▶ The nearest swimming pool is usually not too far away
- ▶ The increased thermal capacity and thermal conductivity of swimming pool water compared to the air leads to an

increased heat supply to the body in the water. Compared to basal metabolic conditions (35°C, complete rest, soberness), the heat dissipation in the water is increased approximately five-fold

▶ Due to the increased heat supply, the metabolic rate of the body rises by 20-100%, to maintain the body temperature, according to the individual fat thickness

▶ With a calorie consumption of 300-600 kcal per hour (depending on swimming style and speed), swimming burns almost as many calories as running, without loading the joints and bones

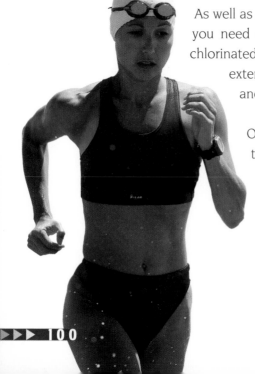

The right Equipment

As well as a bathing suit or swimming trunks, you need chlorine or swimming goggles. In chlorinated water, they protect the sensitive external part of the eyes from irritation and improve visibility in the water.

Outside the pool, it is a good idea to wear bathing shoes to avoid infection from athlete's foot.

The correct Technique

There are four swimming techniques: breaststroke, front crawl, backstroke and butterfly. The latter is not appropriate as an endurance sport for recreational athletes. Whichever technique you eventually choose is up to you. In most cases, people choose the technique they enjoy most and find easiest. If you have back problems, you should get your doctor's opinion on which technique is most suitable for you.

Usually either the front crawl or backstroke are preferred, as in breaststroke the cervical and lumbar spine is permanently overextended (hyperlordosis). There is plenty of literature already available on swimming techniques.

Training Tips

The optimal water temperature for training lies between 26-28°C. If the water is too cold, there is a danger of getting too cold quickly, whereas if the water is too hot (above 28°), heat dissipation can be reduced under high physical loading, resulting in hyperthermia or circulation overload. To stop the body's temperature from rising too high, the body reacts by rerouting the blood circulation from the center of the body to the peripheries. This constitutes a serious circulation overload, though, and heated pools are not intended for swimmers but for relaxation instead.

The last big meal should be eaten 1-2 hours before swimming. In this time, the body is busy supplying blood for digestion, which means there is not enough blood supply left for the muscles used for swimming. Don't jump into the pool overheated from training, but take a shower first.

▶ FAT BURNING

The motto better long and slow than short and fast is as true for swimming as it is for running. It is also basically makes more sense to increase the training duration than the training speed. In the initial training sessions, decide to swim a certain distance, e.g., 500-800 m. It doesn't matter how fast you swim your chosen distance.

It is better to swim calmly and slowly and stop for a short rest after every length to start with, then after every third or fourth length. If you are able, alternate several swimming styles, thus using different muscle groups. After a few training sessions, you can divide the total training distance (e.g., 1000 m) into intervals (e.g., 100 m warm-up; 4 x 100 m breast stroke; 4 x 100 m back stroke; 100 m cool down).

After a few weeks, you should try to swim longer distances without stopping (e.g., 3 x 300 m or 2 x 500 m). Only if you feel fit enough should you now increase your training time from 20-30 minutes to 40-50 minutes.

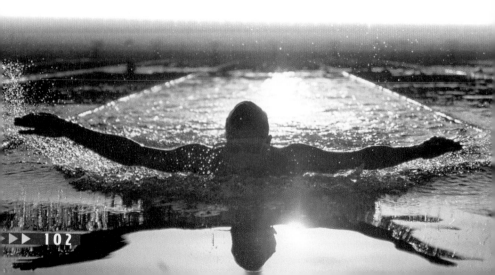

6.4 Cycling

It doesn't matter whether you train on a city bike, a mountain bike or a racing bike. Cycling is healthy for several reasons, particularly for the overweight, and among the specific benefits are:

▶ Cycling is extremely easy on the joints
▶ You are always outside in the fresh air
▶ The training intensity can be optimally measured
▶ For many people, cycling has a high sensation value, which is good for motivation
▶ It develops the cardiovascular system, breathing and metabolism
▶ Cycling can be done at any age

The right Equipment

The range of bicycles available is extremely wide: city bikes, touring bikes, trekking bikes, mountain bikes and racing bikes.

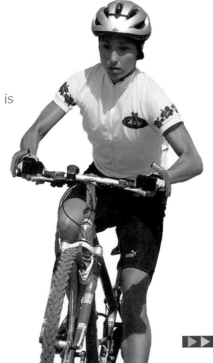

Table 18: Different types of bicycle

City bike	▶ A bicycle for the city
	▶ Comfortable sitting position (more upright than bent over)
	▶ Three, four or seven-speed hub gear
	▶ Good for carrying bags, often 26-inch wheels, wide tires
Touring bike	▶ A very classic bicycle
	▶ Easy to steer, no gears or three-speed hub gear
	▶ 26- or 28-inch wheels with medium-width tires
	▶ The typical Dutch bicycle is also included in this category
Trekking bike	▶ Sporty bicycle for cycling tours
	▶ Sporty frame geometry, inclined sitting position
	▶ Wheels at least 28 inches with medium-width tires
	▶ 24-speed chain gear or seven-speed hub gear
Mountain bike	▶ For use off-road
	▶ Relatively small frame, often with unusual geometry
	▶ At least 26-inch wheels with big-studded tires
	▶ Off-road models lack safety features required by the Highway Code
	▶ 24-speed chain gear with wide gear transmission ratio
Racing bike	▶ Sporty road bike
	▶ Built for speed and extremely light
	▶ 26- or 28-inch wheels with very thin tires
	▶ 21-28-speed chain gear

Training Tips

It is important for training that the bicycle is correctly set up: saddle height and angle, saddle to handlebar distance and, of course, the handlebar height.

- ▶ The saddle should be neither too high nor too low. A simple test is to sit on the saddle, turn one pedal to its lowest point and place the heel on it. The leg should be straight but not overextended.
- ▶ The angle of the saddle is normally horizontal, but this can vary according to individual preference.
- ▶ The distance between the saddle and the handlebars should be such that the knees do not touch the elbows.
- ▶ The handlebars are usually the same height as the saddle. The more sporty your riding style, the lower the handlebars can be, but they should never more than 3-4 cm lower than the saddle.

Training beginners should ride for 20-30 minutes without stopping about three times a week. A previously arduous circuit should become noticeably easier after a few weeks. At this point, the training duration can be increased gradually up to 50-60 minutes.

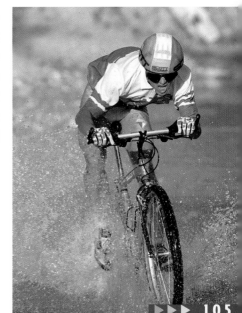

The pedaling rate is an important loading parameter. To be able to ride as far as possible without getting prematurely tired, you should choose a relatively high pedaling rate and a low gear. A pedaling rate of about 90 revolutions per minute has proved to be suitable for most recreational cyclists. Many riders are initially unaccustomed to this high number of revolutions. At this point you should concentrate on a quiet riding style and try not to wobble about too much.

There are bike computer accessories on the market that can show your pedaling rate. It is cheaper just to count your own pedaling rate for one minute and then try to maintain that frequency. You will get a better feel for the right pedaling rate with time.

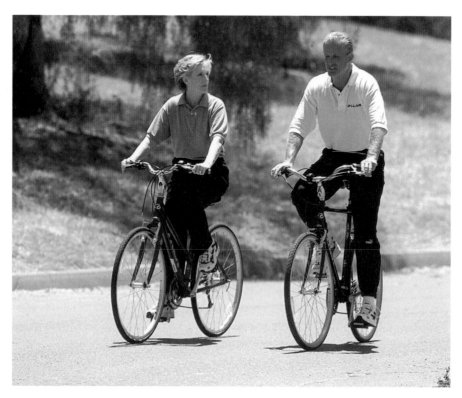

6.5 Inline Skating

A very popular new sport is inline skating, whose participants now run into millions. The great advantages that have led to this boom and made inline skating an ideal endurance sport for weight loss are:

▶ Low, selective loading of the ankles, knees or spinal vertebrae
▶ Even overweight people can carry out high training volumes
▶ Improvement of general aerobic basic endurance and increased metabolic efficiency
▶ Appreciated by many people during hot weather due to the cooling air flow
▶ All in all an optimal endurance sport for weight reduction

The right Gear

A typical inline skate for general fitness training consists of *boot*, *frame* and *wheels*. There are dozens of different kinds of wheels, with varying diameter, hardness, shape and core. Fitness skates are characterized by their comfort and are also relatively fast depending on the price.

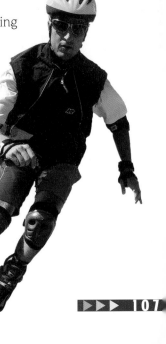

A pair of fitness skates costs from $ 120/ £65 to $ 380/£200. Most skates are also equipped with a brake. Braking systems like ABT from Rollerblades are especially suited to beginners as the whole skate can still touch the ground during the braking process. The braking foot is pushed forward, which triggers a mechanism that drops the brake rubber onto the ground. Others have a sort of back brake that works when the body weight is transferred onto the rear wheels.

The diameter of fitness skate wheels is usually 72-76 mm. ABEC 3 (ABEC = Annular Bearing Engineers Committee, the standard for ball bearings; scale of 1-9) ball bearings are usually recommended by fitness skate manufactures.

Speed skates are only advisable for very advanced skaters. The characteristic of speed skates is that they have five wheels - making them faster but less flexible - and no brake.

Table 19: Fitness and Speed Skates

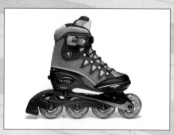

Fitness Skates			
Wheel diameter	Wheel hardness	Ball bearing quality	Price
72-76 mm	78-90 A	ABEC 3-5	£ 70-200

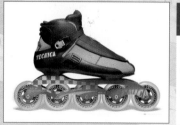

Speed Skates			
Wheel diameter	Wheel hardness	Ball bearing quality	Price
Ca. 80 mm	75-93 A	ABEC 5 and more	£ 140-35•

Tipp

Purchasing tips

▶ The shoes must be comfortable

▶ They must fit without pressing right from the start

▶ Try on with thin socks

▶ Buy in the afternoon after the feet have swelled up a little

▶ The correct fit is more important than the type of bearings

▶ The wheels must roll in a straight line

▶ For beginners, ball bearings of ABEC quality 1-3 are sufficient

▶ Ball bearings that are too fast are not recommended for beginners, as they can be dangerous. It is better to buy faster bearings later on

The minimum safety equipment for inline skating consists of helmet and elbow, knee and wrist guards. But sunglasses and flashing light wheels can also prevent accidents and injuries.

The correct Technique

The basic techniques that a fitness skater should master include the forward skating technique, along with the basic position and the different falling and braking techniques. Beginners should start by practicing the basic position and the different falling and braking techniques and then, as they learn the actual skating technique, practice braking suddenly or, if necessary, also falling without hurting or injuring themselves.

Basic Position

The first steps on inline skates are always difficult. Before learning actual skating techniques, you should be able to adopt a safe but active basic position right from the start. There are several basic positions, which differ in the position of the skates relative to each other. The skates can be parallel to each other (parallel position), placed one behind the other (braking or stopping position), or in the v-position.

The latter is easiest to learn and is usually preferred by beginners. The feet are placed shoulder-width apart in a slight v-position with the heels pointing toward each other. The ankle, knee, and hip joints are slightly bent, the arms are held sideways-forward with the elbows bent and the upper body leaning forward slightly. The head is upright and the eyes look forward. From this basic position, the skater can carry out all other techniques, such as starting, skating and falling.

Where to skate

In the UK and the USA, inline skaters are subject to the same regulations as other road users, i.e., cyclists and car drivers, so these laws should be respected. Always give way to pedestrians when skating on pavements or public footpaths.

Falling Techniques

Falls are common in skating, most of which are without serious consequences. To avoid pain and injury when falling, the inline skater must not only wear suitable protection but also make an effort to learn and practice falling from the start.

The skater must get used to the ground. While when you fall from running, you try not to land on the joints, when skating one deliberately uses the joints to bounce from as they are protected. The techniques are different for falling forward, sideways and backward.

Both when falling backward and sideways, try to turn very fast so that you face forward and falls forward, thus reducing the risk of injury. While this is relatively easy when falling to the side, a half-turn around the body's axis when falling backward is more difficult to pull off.

Try to absorb the impact of the fall with the *wrist guards*, with the fingers spread and the impulse absorbed or reduced by the arms. This is the only way to avoid a painful landing on the bottom or back.

In the first phase of the forward fall, try to fall onto the knee pads once you have lowered your center of gravity. The hips are now blocked, the back is kept straight and the arms are held out to the side with the fingers spread out. Only then should you fall onto the elbow pads, keeping the head up. The palms of the hand face forward with the fingers still spread out.

In the last phase, the momentum is reduced still further, where the skater falls on the wrist guards and carries the momentum onto the ground, if possible. During this last phase, it is important to tuck the head into the neck and draw the lower leg into the bottom. All three protected joints are now touching the ground.

Watch points for the correct forward-falling technique:

▶ Lower the body's center of gravity!
▶ First, fall onto your knees!
▶ Then, onto your elbows!
▶ Finally, onto your hands!

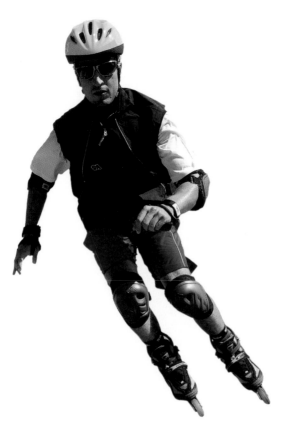

The correct Way to stand up

Standing up in the right way should also be learned right at the start, in combination with the falling technique. If you feel very unsure on your skates to begin with, try standing up on the grass or use a fence or railing for help.

- ▶ Kneel so that both knee guards touch the ground, and support yourself with both hands
- ▶ Place one foot flat on the ground next to the knee of the other leg
- ▶ Place both hands on the knee
- ▶ Start to stand up slowly and draw in the other foot
- ▶ Only then straighten the upper body
- ▶ Adopt a stable basic position

Be careful not to lean too far forward when you stand up, as this will make the skates roll backward.

Starting

After the first skating basics have been learned – basic position, falling and standing up – the real skating can start. Always start from a position in which the legs are at an angle of 40-60% to each other. One skate is placed slightly forward, while the rear skate is placed slightly diagonally behind it. Bend the legs slightly, look forward and the transfer the body weight mainly over the front foot.

When you actually start, push off from the inside of the rear skate and extend the rear leg back out to the side. This extending pushing movement brings the body weight almost completely onto the front leg and you will start to glide. The rear leg is then brought back under the body and, after a short gliding phase, what was formerly the front leg now becomes the push-off leg.

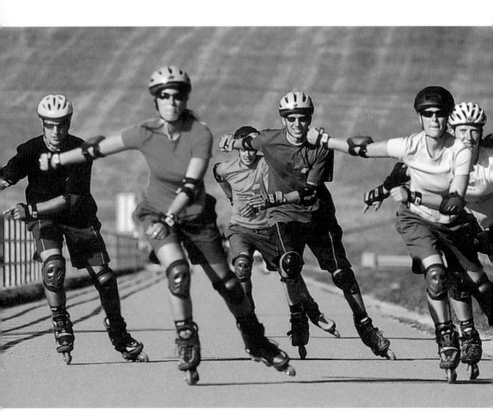

Braking Techniques

The simplest mechanical braking techniques are the heel stop and the T stop. To learn braking techniques, start with a few strokes to get going and then adopt a parallel basic position and try to perform one of the braking techniques. Start slowly and gradually build up speed. The mechanical braking techniques are the most important for the fitness skater.

Table 20: Braking techniques

Heel Stop	▶ Push the braking foot forward and adopt the step position
	▶ Press both hands on the thigh of the front leg
	▶ Bend the support leg and lower the body's center of gravity
	▶ Raise the toe area until the brake block touches the ground
	▶ Extend the braking and leading leg to increase the braking pressure
T-Stop	▶ Shift the weight onto the front leg
	▶ Bend the knees slightly and lean the upper body forward
	▶ Bend the arms and hold them to the front
	▶ Turn the rear skate and place it at an angle of 90° to the skating direction
	▶ Lightly drag the inside of the rear skate along the ground
	▶ Increase the braking effect by bending the front leg

Forward Skating Technique

After the basic inline skating skills have been learned, you can now begin to learn to skate forward. This includes basic rhythm skating, curve skating and the crossover.

Table 21: Forward skating techniques

Basic Rhythm	▶ Fluent, cyclical action between pushing off and gliding
	▶ After the start position there is a powerful extending movement from the inside of the rear skate onto the front gliding leg
	▶ The gliding leg touches the ground with the outside edge of the skate
	▶ During the ensuing gliding phase, the opposite arm swings forward and the rear leg is brought out and then placed in front of the other leg.
	▶ Bend the upper body and the knees slightly face forward
Curve Skating	▶ Two-legged gliding forward
	▶ Take the step position (the foot nearest the bend is in front)
	▶ The body weight is over the outside edge of the skate nearest the curve and the inside edge of the outer skate
	▶ Lower the body's center of gravity
	▶ The shoulder nearest the curve is turned inward
	▶ Look in the direction of the curve
Cross-over (Left curve)	▶ The body weight is over the outside edge of the bent left leg (nearest the curve)
	▶ The right leg is placed behind (step position), with the weight on the inside edge
	▶ Push and straighten the right leg
	▶ Transfer all body weight onto the outside edge of the left leg
	▶ Lift the right skate and cross it over in front of the left skate
	▶ Transfer body weight onto the right skate
	▶ Lift the unloaded left skate and then tuck it in front of the right skate
	▶ The upper body leans strongly into the curve
	▶ The inside shoulder turns slightly inward; the arm points to the center of the circle

Training tips

▶ Start with technique training
▶ Next find a car-free and flat training area
▶ Never skate without protection
▶ Skate with your back as straight as possible
▶ Respect the rules of the Highway Code
▶ Vary training forms (interval methods, Fartlek)
▶ Always warm up and cool down
▶ First increase training duration and then intensity
▶ Better to train longer and slower than fast and short

6.6 Cross-country Skiing

Cross-country skiing, an ancient mode of winter transport, is now considered to be the optimal winter endurance sport par excellence and is actually one of the healthiest of all sports.

Cross-country skiing features a gliding, low-impact action in the fresh clear winter air in a snowy landscape.

One disadvantage of cross-country skiing is that it is a seasonal sport. The specific advantages of cross-country skiing are:

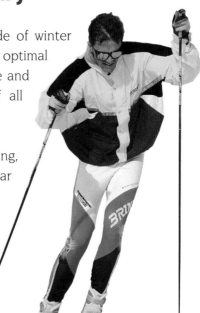

▶ In principle, recommended for all age groups
▶ As a low-impact sport with a gliding action, it is especially suitable for the overweight
▶ It is whole-body training, soliciting large muscle groups in both the upper and lower body
▶ As a result, there is also a very high metabolic demand. Depending on intensity, cross-country skiing can burn 400-1000 kcal per hour

Cross-country Skiing Equipment

Cross-country skis have no blades, unlike downhill skis, and are about 45-50 mm wide. The better your technique, the narrower your skis should be. The length of the skis depends mainly on your height, the type of ski and your body weight.

They are normally about 10-30 cm longer than one's height. Skating skis are usually a little shorter than a classic diagonal ski. Body weight also influences the choice of ski length:

▶ The heavier the skier, the longer the ski should be
▶ The lighter the skier, the shorter the ski should be

There are two types of skis: diagonal and skating skis. If you want to use the classic diagonal stride and double stick push in a sprinting cross-country ski run, choose a diagonal ski.

There are also two types of diagonal ski: waxable or waxless. The push-off zone of the no-wax ski has "fish scales" or fine artificial hairs on the surface and must not be worked with glide wax. A waxable ski has a completely smooth surface and must be waxed before every run, depending on the snow conditions.

Waxable skis are mainly used by advanced skiers as the waxing preparation requires a lot of experience.

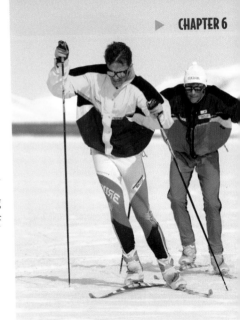

The paper strip test for diagonal skiers

The push-off zone is in the center of the diagonal ski. This only touches the ground during the push-off itself. Use the paper strip test to check whether only the front and back part of the ski really touch the ground. Take the ski and then find its center of gravity by balancing it on your index finger. The push-off zone extends over 1.5 feet in front of and 1 foot behind the center of gravity. Now place both skis on a surface that is a flat as possible (a flat floor or a large table). Stand with the tips of both feet on the center of gravity on the skis (this is how you stand on the skis when the binding is fixed). If the skis are suitable for your body weight, a leaf of paper can be passed under the skis, but if you shift your weight onto one ski, the paper should be stuck to the floor.

The skating ski is somewhat shorter and stiffer than the diagonal ski and is used with the ice-skating or skating technique. Like the downhill ski, the bottom surface is completely smooth.

The skating ski should not be too soft as this makes it too slow and, at the push-off, the middle of the ski is pushed down too far into the snow. Too hard a skating ski is not fast either, as this is hard to control on a side push-off and the blade of the ski sinks into the snow.

Cross-country bindings and sticks are also part of the equipment. Cross-country bindings allow a rolling motion of the foot while the toes are fixed, and adequate ski control is guaranteed (diagonal binding), whereas in a skating binding, the heel is held as near as possible to the ski.

Cross country poles are made of light metal, fiberglass, carbon or other carbon compounds. The price is mainly determined by the quality. Many cross country beginners use poles that are too long, making the learning process more difficult.

▶ Sticks for the classic technique: height minus 30 cm (shoulder height)
▶ Sticks for the skating technique: height minus 20 cm (chin height)

When buying cross-country ski boots, bear in mind that you should not buy the cheapest but the ones that fit the best. Only an optimal fit can prevent rubbing and blisters. Good cross-country boots have a soft but very effective heel binding.

Cross-country Techniques

Cross-country skiing techniques are relatively complex. The two most popular are the diagonal technique and the skating technique. Others are the walking, double stick push and various braking techniques.

The technique descriptions are quite long-winded, so for more information, consult the appropriate literature.

6.7 Walking

"Walking is the best medicine." This is not a new idea, as this quotation comes from the Greek doctor and philosopher Socrates, who impressed his fellow men 2,400 years ago.

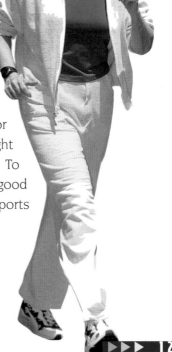

Walking is a low-impact sport comparable with inline skating and, at the right intensity, it is the best sport for weight reduction.

Endurance walking is particularly suitable for people with joint problems and the overweight and is better for these groups than jogging. To take up walking, all you need are a pair of good walking or jogging shoes and some suitable sports clothes. The specific benefits of walking are:

- ▶ Outdoor sport
- ▶ Can be done almost anywhere
- ▶ Quick to learn
- ▶ Low impact
- ▶ No injury risk
- ▶ Very cheap

The correct Technique

Walking is technically different both from everyday walking and race walking, which is an athletics event. The most important movement features of walking include:

- ▶ Upright, relaxed and deliberate action
- ▶ Arms bent at 90° swing at the side of the body
- ▶ Vigorous arm action
- ▶ Hands are relaxed or form a fist
- ▶ Alternate arm and leg action (right leg, left arm)
- ▶ The upper body remains as still as possible
- ▶ Shoulders hang loosely
- ▶ Deliberate rolling foot motion from heel to toe
- ▶ One foot should always have contact with the ground

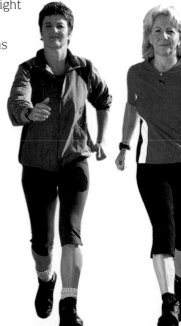

Important aspects of walking are also speed and stride rate. Both are far higher than that of everyday walking. Whereas in walking, one trains at speeds of 3 –5km/h with about 100-120 strides per minute, the intensity of power or race walking is far higher.

Here, the tempo is about 9km/h, and the stride rate is well over 100 strides per minute. The cardiovascular load is naturally also correspondingly higher. Also, the type of route (hills, sand) and the distance have an effect on the demand. The faster you walk, the shorter the strides and the higher the stride rate.

	Speed	Stride Rate
Strolling	1.5-3km/h	40-45 strides/minute
Walking	3-5km/h	100-120 strides/minute
Power walking	5-9km/h	120-150 strides/minute

Variations of Walking

Along with the traditional form of walking, there are also the following alternatives: power walking, hill walking, Nordic walking, snow walking and wogging.

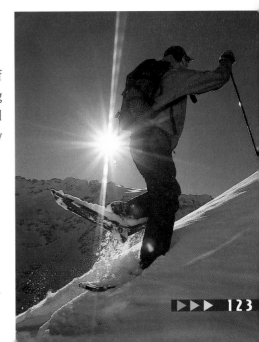

Snow Walking

Table 22: Different types of walking

Power Walking	▶ Fast walking at 5-9 km/h
	▶ Initial training with the extensive interval method
Hill Walking	▶ Hill-walking (= walking uphill), increased training demand
	▶ Not for beginners and inexperienced walkers
	▶ Downhill walking puts increased strain on joints
Nordic Walking	▶ Dynamic walking with specially developed sticks
	▶ 20-30% more effective than walking without sticks
	▶ Particularly suitable for people with knee and back problems as there is 30% less stress on the locomotor system.
Snow Walking	▶ A new version of snow-shoe walking
	▶ Walking in the snow with half-meter-long oval boards
	▶ Very exciting, but also very arduous
Wogging	▶ For experienced walkers
	▶ Loading can be increased by small dumbbells or wrist or underarm weights
	▶ Strengthening of the upper body, shoulder and arm muscles
	▶ Increased calorie consumption

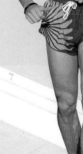

6.8 Aqua Jogging

Aqua jogging is the most suitable endurance sport for the overweight, as it is non-weight bearing. Aqua jogging is becoming more established alongside the traditional endurance sports of running, swimming, cycling, cross-country skiing and walking. Aqua jogging stands out compared to these other endurance sports due to a range of specific benefits:

- ▶ Low impact cardiovascular training
- ▶ High energy metabolism/calorie consumption
- ▶ Low injury risk

These advantages and the specific effects of the water on the human body make aqua jogging optimally suited for losing weight. Among the specific advantages of exercising in water are:

- ▶ More economical heart activity
- ▶ Relief of the joints and ligaments
- ▶ Stimulation of the metabolism
- ▶ Physical and mental relaxation

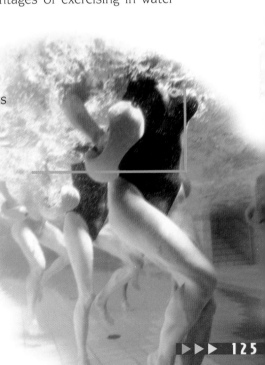

Metabolism

Aqua jogging provides exceptional stimulation for the energy metabolism. As well as the basic stimulation of the energy metabolism by the coldness of the water (provided that the water is colder than 33°C), aqua jogging utilizes a relatively high percentage of skeletal musculature.

The fat metabolism in particular can be specifically trained by aqua jogging, when the raised basal metabolic rate in the water leads to the glycogen reserves being depleted more rapidly and the fat metabolism takes over earlier as the dominant energy supply.

The metabolism is also raised for a longer amount of time after training due to the water's cooling effect on the body. All these effects combined can bring about lasting weight loss. At 38 strides/minute (a very low load), in 1992, Michaud, Sherman & Brennan established an average calorie consumption of 222 kcal (929J) per hour for women and 327 kcal (1,369J) per hour for men. Research at the University of Virginia has even been able to establish a calorie demand of up to 1,000 kcal per hour compared to 600-800 kcal per house for running.

Development of Aqua Jogging

Glen MacWaters, the athletics coach of the U.S. Marines, carried out his own rehabilitation in the water after a foot injury back in 1970. In the 1980s, he developed the WetVest® so that he could carry out running specific training during rehabilitation.

It has been used by many top American athletes since the early '80s, the most well-known of whom was the world-class athlete Mary Decker-Slaney, who suffered a painful Achilles tendon injury just a few weeks before the Olympic Games of 1984.

After 17 days' intensive water running training, she still managed to take part in the Olympic Games and, just after resuming normal training, she set a world 2,000 m record.

The right Equipment

As water running without buoyancy aids is very uncontrolled and leads to swimming-type movements, it is best to use an Aquajogger®, which provides just enough buoyancy so that running movement can be carried out without auxiliary swimming movements. Aquajoggers® are available in different buoyancy levels and sizes and can even be made to measure.

Buoyancy vests cost between $ 30/£15 and $ 60/£30 depending on the product. Some manufacturers offer additional accessories for aqua jogging training, which are mainly intended to increase the overall training intensity or the demand on specific muscle groups. Such accessories are:

- ► Ankle weights
- ► Dumbbell-shaped buoyancy aids
- ► Gloves

The correct Technique

There are two types of running in water: (a) running while touching the bottom of the pool, known as water running, which is carried out in shallow water, and (b) running in water without touching the bottom, known as deep water running, which is carried out exclusively in deep water. In general, aqua jogging refers to the second type. There are four main techniques: running, striding, high knees and the robo jog technique. The latter, in particular, is used mainly for rehabilitation.

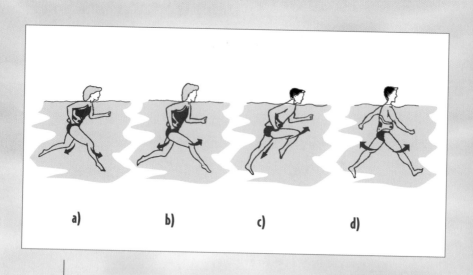

Figure 9: Aqua jogging techniques: a) running, b) striding, c) high-knee running d) robo jog

Before starting to run, an orthopeaedically sound running posture should be adopted, with the following features:

- ▶ Slight forward lean
- ▶ Head up
- ▶ Extension of the thoracic vertebrae
- ▶ Elbow angle of 90°

The vigorous arm action from the shoulders is the same for all four running techniques. The running technique is like a combination of running and cycling and is principally characterized by a forward swing of the lower leg and the extension backward of the legs.

The main movement feature of the striding run is the wide amplitude of the strides. High-knee running is characterized by the alternate raising of the knees to a horizontal position at high speed and with an active extension backward and downward of the legs. The legs are always kept straight during the robo jog.

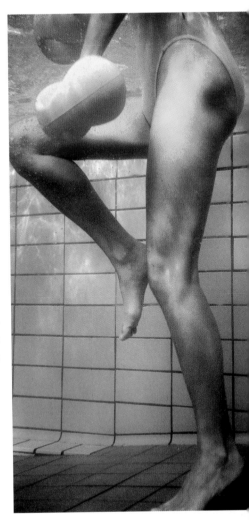

Table 23: The main features of the four aqua jogging techniques:

Running
- ▶ The spine is extended
- ▶ The hands are loosely closed or flattened
- ▶ The lower leg swings forward
- ▶ The legs are swung backward
- ▶ The arms swing at an angle of 90° from the shoulders
- ▶ No "swimming" arm action
- ▶ The feet swing loosely and firmly sideways and forward
- ▶ Stride rate: 25:45 strides/minute

Striding
- ▶ Extend the feet forward
- ▶ Extend the toes forward
- ▶ Straighten the legs right back
- ▶ Bring the knees up higher than for normal running
- ▶ Arm swing is greater and more vigorous than for step running
- ▶ Stride rate: 20-30 strides/minute

High-Knees Running
- ▶ Lift the knees alternately to above hip height
- ▶ Active downward and backward extension of the legs
- ▶ No lower leg swing
- ▶ Stride rate: 30-60 strides/min

Robo jog
- ▶ Legs are completely straight
- ▶ Arm angle varies
- ▶ Toes are raised as legs are brought forward
- ▶ Stride rate: 15-30 strides/minute

Aqua Jogging Training

Aqua jogging is most suitable for training the cardiovascular system. It can also be great for training strength endurance, mobility or coordination, depending on the motor deficit available. Aqua jogging is an optimal endurance training method, as it is the ideal combination of the positive aspects of training in water with those of endurance training.

Whichever training method is used depends on the fitness of the individual and the training goal. If the aim is to lose weight, aqua jogging must mainly be done as endurance training, i.e., long sessions at low intensity.

The endurance method with a loading of 60-70% is the obvious method of choice. The session should last at least 30 minutes. It can also be alternated with the extensive interval method with long intervals (5 – 10 mins). Such training sessions should be carried out 2-3 times per week.

In aqua jogging, too, training sessions should be divided into three phases: warm-up, workout and cool-down. The *warm-up* can consist of e.g., aquagym, slow running, and stretching. In the *workout*, endurance training is the focus. Strengthening, coordination and mobility exercises can also be integrated into sessions.

The *cool-down* phase can either be active (games, slow running) or passive exercise or relaxation forms (stretching, relaxation). In aqua relaxation (relaxation in water), the aim is to intensify the relaxation effect by closing the eyes. Appropriate music and mentally "shifting inside oneself" in pleasant surroundings can enhance feelings of relaxation.

6.9 Spinning®

Spinning® means cycling on special stationary bikes (Spinning® Bikes), following the specific loading instructions of a trained Spinning® instructor. In most cases, the training is carried out to appropriate lively music that simulates a bicycle ride. Spinning® is perfect training for anyone who wants a fast improvement in endurance and strength endurance, especially in the leg muscles. However, it is not only suitable for improving the conditioning ability of the cardiovascular system, but also as training for deliberate weight reduction.

Spinning® is not just a great training method for cyclists, runners and triathletes, it also provides an optimal start to endurance training for the large group of fitness athletes, false beginners, those with joint problems and the overweight. Every athlete can set their own resistance level and therefore their own load. This individual loading control makes it possible for

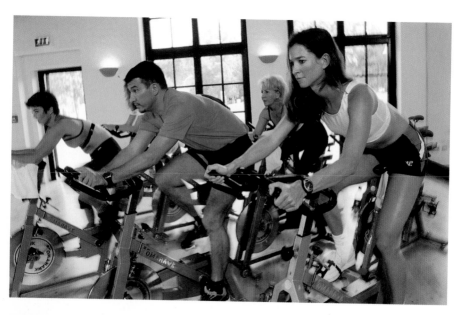

an experienced cyclist and a recreational athlete to take part in the same class. The intensity regulation takes place without scaling, so that there is no danger of the pointless ambition of beating your neighbor. Recreational and health training goals can be achieved if you monitor your heart rate and follow the teacher's instructions.

JOHNNY G – The Inventor of Spinning®

As the inventor of this modern, low-impact form of endurance training, Jonathan Goldberg, this professional South African racing cyclist and extreme endurance athlete, is known as Johnny G for short. In his preparation for the hardest marathon cycle race in the world, the *Race Across America* (RAAM), he was looking for ways to do part of his training indoors. He created an extensive training program that he continually improved upon.

Johnny G built a stationary bike in his garage, which he used to do his indoor training. He equipped his bike with a special fly wheel. He called the training program Spinning® because of the self-turning flywheel (spin the wheel). It was not long before the first group training took place in his garage in Los Angeles. He played music to increase training motivation.

This innovative and trendy type of group training drew larger and larger crowds and soon the first training sessions were taking place in gyms in Santa Monica and Los Angeles. In 1989, the first Johnny G Spinning® Center was opened in Santa Monica, California.

Today, Spinning® is practiced worldwide in over 100 countries and 75,000 instructors have already been trained. ("Johnny G Spinning® "R" Certificate").

In the meantime, many other forms of Spinning® have sprung up alongside Johnny G's, which is the source of all the other variations. Fitness experts and industry connoisseurs agree that the popularity of Spinning® in all its forms will not stop growing in the years to come.

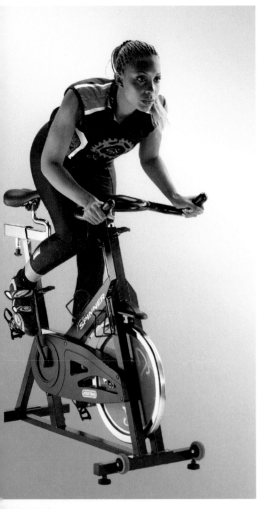

Benefits of Spinning®

From physical, mental and social points of view, Spinning® possesses a variety of benefits and actually counts as one of the best endurance sports.

By changing the sitting position and handlebar grip, the upper-body muscles can be strengthened, as well as the legs. The pedal resistance is continuously adjustable and can be changed to simulate cycling uphill or downhill. The main benefits of Spinning® are as follows:

▶ The joint loading during Spinning® is extremely low
▶ No difficult coordination abilities or movement patterns are required
▶ You can start to do complicated techniques directly in training without a long learning phase
▶ The resistance can be adjusted to suit each individual
▶ Athletes of all ages and fitness levels can train together
▶ The group atmosphere is extremely motivating
▶ Strengthening of the leg, arm and shoulder muscles
▶ It is fun, extremely motivating and helps to get a second wind to move in time to stimulating music
▶ Rain, snow and cold are irrelevant. No flat tires either!

Danger of Overloading

According to a report in a medical journal, Spinning® can present a danger of overloading for certain target groups. Spinning®, in its typical form as basic endurance or fat-burning training, is not suitable for the unfit, the elderly and those with cardiovascular problems. The music and the encouragement of the instructor make physical overloading and training at too high an intensity a danger, hence the need for (a) a prior medical check-up and (b) training at a moderate level.

The danger of overloading exists in Spinning®, as in running and other endurance sports. A well-trained Spinning® instructor knows of this danger and tries to make his less-fit clients train at a lower intensity. Spinning® training at an appropriately low load adapted for the target group is more suitable for the improvement of general aerobic endurance rather than for weight reduction by fat burning.

The Spinning® Bike

Compared to the conventional bicycle and gym bikes, which have an idling cycle, the Spinning® bike is equipped with a so-called star gear, whereby the bottom bracket and flywheel are directly coupled together. This type of gear makes Spinning® particularly attractive, but some people can find it a little strange at first. It is important to set the saddle and handlebar heights, and the distance between the saddle and handlebars correctly to provide an optimal sitting position.

Johnny developed special stationary bikes suitable for mass production, called *Spinning® Bikes*, in connection with the American company Schwinn. But other companies have also joined the trend and developed similar stationary bikes without an idling cycle and with a large flywheel. The bikes possess a continuously adjustable brake, so that the resistance can be adjusted according to one's fitness. Spinning® Bikes either have toe cages or clipless pedals. Unlike the gym bike, it has no computer display to show the loading level or pedaling rate.

The correct Technique

The most important Spinning® techniques are pedaling, and the different grips and riding positions.

The technique of an inexperienced cyclist is characterized by a jerky and inefficient action, where the only effective power is generated in the pushing phase. So, years ago, the circular pedaling action was invented, in which feet and legs move in a fluent and synchronized movement on a circular path. As in cycle racing, the pedaling action in Spinning® should be as "round" as possible, as this is the only way to make the most of the whole circular action.

This gives an optimal workout for the hamstring and quad muscles, as well as the calves and the buttocks. Try to keep the rest of the body still as you pedal, particularly the upper body, which should not wobble about. The legs move parallel to the frames and the knees face forward. To summarize, a good technique is characterized by the following movement features:

- ► Quiet upper body
- ► Parallel leg action
- ► Loose and circular pedaling action

From a technical point of view, pedaling is a riding technique in which the pedal is not only pushed downward, but backward in the lower pedal position and forward in the upper position.

With racing pedals, there is also a very powerful backward and upward pull. So, pedaling can be split into four phases:

Table 24: Pedaling phases

Phase	Position	Technique	Musculature
Pushing phase	1-5 o'clock	Push down vertically on the pedal. Phase of greatest power transfer.	▶ quadriceps ▶ calf muscles
Gliding phase	5-7 o'clock	Transition from the pushing phase to the pulling phase.	
Pulling phase	7-10 o'clock	A half-way foot extension pulls the leg upward and backward. The toes are lowered, the heels raised (recovery phase for the rectus femoris).	▶ shin muscles ▶ hamstrings
Dynamic pushing phase "squaring the circle"	10-1 o'clock	In this phase, the foot is pushed forward, and the heels are lowered.	▶ shin muscles ▶ hip flexors

Fluent pedaling also requires as even as possible a driving action from both legs. Most sportspeople have a dominant leg. This can have a variety of causes:

- ▶ Unbalanced training
- ▶ Difference in leg length
- ▶ Previous injuries

Here is a test to establish whether there is a difference in driving power between your legs:

Pedal for three minutes against the same resistance and at the same rate first with the right leg and then with the left (this may be repeated several times according to training condition).

The dominant leg will tire noticeably later than the weaker one

According to the pedaling technique chosen, the sportsperson should adopt a suitable handlebar grip. In Spinning®, there are three main alternatives:

▶ Narrow grip: hands are placed on the handle bar
▶ Wide grip: hands are placed on the angle of the handle bar
▶ Aggressive grip: hands grip the ends of the handlebar

To make training as motivating and varied as possible, you should learn different riding positions so that you work different muscle groups.

Table 25: Riding positions

Riding in the sitting position	▶ Narrow grip ▶ Basic Spinning® technique
Climbing from sitting position	▶ Wide grip ▶ Increased resistance (uphill) ▶ Bottom shifted backward a little ▶ Drive by both legs as equally as possible
Riding from standing position	▶ Wide grip ▶ Average resistance ▶ Rhythmic pedaling action
Climbing from standing position	▶ Aggressive grip ▶ Higher resistance (only for the advanced) ▶ Body's center of gravity over the pedals ▶ Marked up and down motion of the body
Bouncing	▶ Wide grip ▶ Standing up and sitting down for a period of time ▶ Fluent transitions ▶ Pedaling rate remains the same
Sprinting in sitting position	▶ Narrow grip ▶ Light resistance ▶ Very high number of revolutions per minute/pedaling rate ▶ Relaxed upper body
Sprinting from standing position	▶ Wide grip ▶ Difficult technique ▶ Very high number of revolutions per minute/ high pedaling rate ▶ Try to keep the body at the same height

Spinning® Training

Spinning® training sessions should also be divided into the classic three phases of warm-up, workout and cool-down. Depending on the intention and training condition of the individual, the duration of the session can vary considerably. Most training sessions last about 45 minutes, but for the very advanced, they can last up to 90 minutes.

The idea is to pedal without stopping and at a high rate, in the sitting and standing positions. The pedaling rate is, on average, between 80-120 revs per minute, and can be more. Professional road cyclists usually travel at rates of 120 revs per minute on the flat.

The principle of a Spinning® session can be compared to a ride through mountains and valleys. Start off slowly in the warm-up phase, i.e., on the plain. A five-minute warm-up is an absolute "must," despite the low risk of injury, as it stimulates the metabolism, which in turn raises the body temperature, activates the cardiovascular and respiratory systems and brings the Spinning®-specific muscles up to an operating temperature.

The first hill appears in the actual workout phase. The resistance is increased noticeably and the pedaling rate decreases. The terrain becomes steeper and steeper, you can get out of the saddle and increase the pressure on the fly-wheel. In a downhill ride, the resistance is substantially reduced, so that the pedaling rate can be increased once again.

At the end of an intensive Spinning® session, there is a relaxing finale, with relaxed, low intensity cycling, followed, of course, by a stretching program for the muscles previously utilized. The warm-down accelerates recovery, prevents muscle soreness and avoids long-term problems (e.g., muscular imbalances, incorrect posture). The duration of the cool-down depends on the target group and especially on the duration and intensity of the preceding workout load.

The Spinning® Program

Johnny G. Spinning® is the most successful group training program in the world and works as an individual or integrated training concept. Workouts are led by a certified Johnny G. Spinning® instructor. The landscape is formed by music and rhythm, which can be simulated perfectly with the aid of a variable resistance regulation on the bike and different riding techniques.

By taking advantage of the positive group dynamic effect, Spinning® offers the possibility of finding one's own individual, goal-oriented energy load in different energy zones. Pulserate-controlled Spinning® training at compensation, basic, development and competition level thus enables almost every target group to reach their desired training goal.

It is the interaction of endurance, strength, technique, speed, mobility and psychological elements that makes the Spinning® program so successful. They are included in every individual training session, through the introduction of specific Spinning® Energy Zones™, which comprise the following areas as measured by the maximal heart rate:

Table 26: Spinning® Energy Zones™

Spinning® Energy Zones™ Loading (HRmax)	
Recovery	50-65%
Endurance	65-75%
Strength	75-85%
Interval	65-92%
Race Day	80-92%

The target group who train to lose weight should train mainly in the *endurance zone*. This corresponds most to the fat-burning zone (60-70% of maximal heart rate). The heart rate in the *endurance zone* is 65-75% of the maximal heart rate, i.e., you should initially train at the lower limit of this zone. Training includes seated riding, on the flat and in the hills.

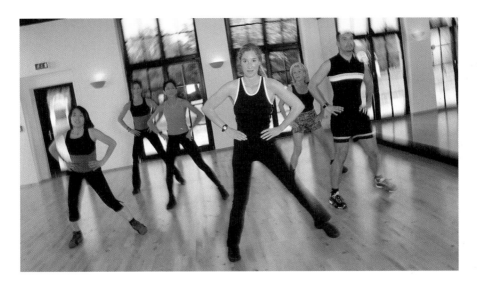

6.10 Hiking

Hiking is not just wandering aimlessly around in the countryside, but can be considered an extremely effective and healthy lifetime sport. Along with developing the physical main demand forms especially endurance and strength, and the coordination abilities (especially balance and reaction abilities), hiking also develops the psychosocial side. And, incidentally, a long hike burns plenty of fat, as the loading volume is high.

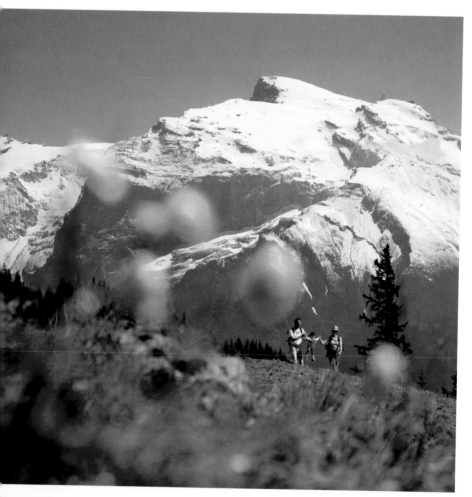

Calorie consumption for hiking

The fluid and energy requirements for mountain walking are relatively high. The calorie requirement is calculated according to the walking distance and the change in altitude:

▶ 1km mountain walking flat	About 50 kcal
▶ Ascent of 100 m altitude	About 100 kcal
▶ Ascent of 100 m altitude in loose snow	About 150 kcal
▶ Descent of 100 m altitude	About 23 kcal
▶ 1 km walking downhill	About 63 kcal

The basal metabolic rate of a person weighing 82kg accounts for about 82 x 25 = 2,050 kcal. The active metabolic rate on a mountain with ascents and descents of 800m of altitude accounts for about 1,000 calories (8 x 100 + 8 x 23). The total calorie requirement (basal rate + active rate) therefore stands at about 3,050 calories. This example shows that on a long mountain walk, 1,500-2,000 calories can be used up in addition to the daily basal rate with no problem at all.

The right Equipment

Above all, mountain walkers need good shoes (trekking shoes) and also functional clothes (cf. Chapter 9), a rucksack and some other accessories.

Solid footwear is by far the most important item of equipment for the mountain walker. *Trekking shoes* are recommended, as their light weight makes climbing a lot easier than traditional climbing boots. Trekking shoes should have the following properties:

▶ High-tops
▶ Stable ankle area
▶ Non-slip, anti-torsion profile rubber sole
▶ Good heel fit
▶ Orthopaedic footbed

To be comfortable, a rucksack must fit close to the body and the larger models should have a belt. The size of the rucksack depends on the length of the mountain hike. A capacity of 20-30 liters is sufficient for a normal hike, but for one lasting several days, a medium-sized rucksack with 50-60 liter capacity is required. It is also an advantage that rucksacks have many external and internal pockets for all the small articles you need on a mountain hike. In particular, interior pockets with integrated map pockets have proved useful.

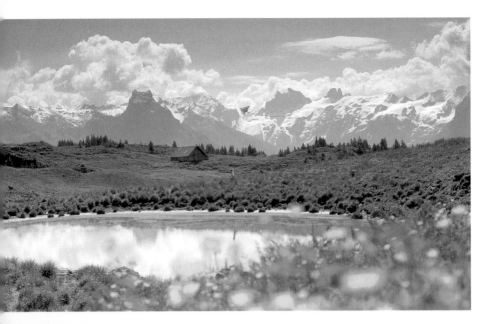

Along with suitable footwear, clothing adapted to hiking and a rucksack, on an all-day mountain hike, you should on no account forget the following items:

- ▶ Telescopic stick
- ▶ Drinking flask and thermos flask
- ▶ Sufficient food (chocolate or muesli bars as back-up)
- ▶ Headgear, rain clothes, sunglasses
- ▶ First-aid kit
- ▶ Up-to-date walking guides and maps (survey maps on a scale of 1:100,000; topographic maps 1:50,000 or 1:25,000)
- ▶ Compass and altimeter (also to be used as a barometer)
- ▶ Safety blanket and signaling whistle
- ▶ Sunscreen lotion and lip protection for a high-altitude hike
- ▶ Penknife

The correct Technique

Hiking is easy to learn, and some people can do it well into old age. The main techniques of hiking, i.e., walking and climbing, are basic acquired human skills.

There are also increased demands in the coordination (balance) and the conditioning areas, where strength endurance in the lower limbs is required along with basic endurance.

While walking and climbing along paths is technically very easy, the techniques in rough terrain (e.g., firn and scree) must be learned.

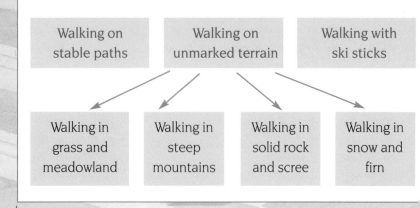

Figure 10: An overview of the most important hiking techniques

A few basic aspects can be formulated for all techniques:

▶ Think about every step you make

▶ Always look a few steps ahead

▶ Adjust your stride length to your height and the gradient

▶ When going up or downhill, take the route of the lowest altitude difference

▶ Place the load as evenly as possible on the sole of your foot

▶ Transfer the body weight onto the support leg so as to maintain balance

▶ Breathe in time with your walking rhythm

Joint Loading

Along with the many sports physiological benefits of hiking, the joint loading, especially on the lower limbs (ankles, knee and hip joints) and the spine, should not be underestimated. There is a particularly high load when walking downhill, where the already high loading is increased even further by the weight of the rucksack.

▶ Wear stable and ankle-high climbing boots

▶ Walk uphill and come down with the ropeway/funicular or chairlift

▶ Use light rucksacks and equipment

▶ Only take with you what you really need

▶ Use ski sticks going downhill and keep them near to the body

▶ Wear joint bandages if you suffer from knee pain

▶ Go slowly downhill with small steps

▶ Climb down big steps, don't jump

▶ Keep your joints warm

▶ Breathe calmly and evenly

If you like the idea of losing weight by hiking regularly, you should read detailed technical descriptions and the following topics beforehand.

- ▶ Preparation for hiking
- ▶ The dangers of mountain weather
- ▶ Orienteering for hikers
- ▶ Emergencies in the mountains

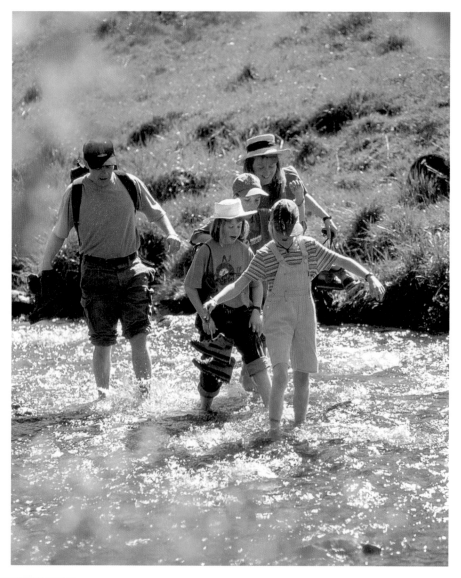

Aerobic Fitness Equipment

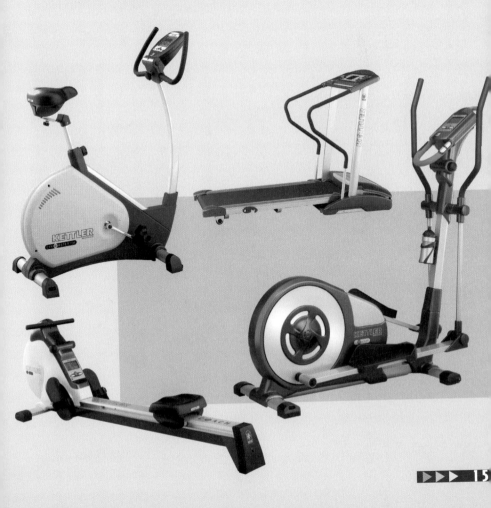

▶ FAT BURNING

Various aerobic fitness trends are just as suitable for weight loss as the endurance sports, in particular the following fitness equipment:

- ▶ Treadmill
- ▶ Rowing machine
- ▶ Cross-trainer
- ▶ Gym bicycle
- ▶ Exercise machine
- ▶ Stepper

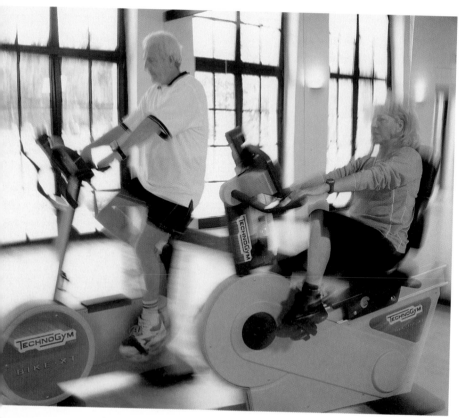

Treadmill Training

Indoor running training on a treadmill has many advantages:

▶ Can be carried out at any time of day, especially in winter
▶ No excuses in bad weather
▶ Quality treadmills have very good shock absorption
▶ No joint problems from running on concrete

A treadmill should be as easy as possible to fold away vertically. A strong engine runs comparatively quietly, and a treadmill with a large running surface makes training more secure. The overweight and people with back or knee problems should only train on a treadmill with extremely good shock-absorbing properties.

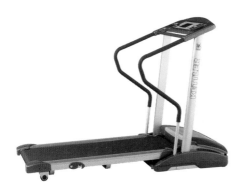

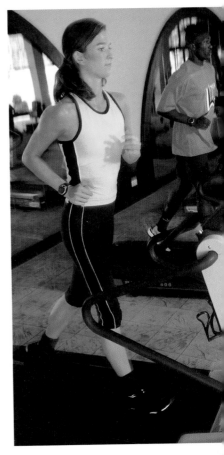

Rowing Machines

Training on a rowing machine is an extremely effective form of cardiovascular training. It strengthens the upper and lower limbs, as well as the trunk muscles. This training is also beneficial for the fat metabolism, as the large muscle groups are utilized by rowing training.

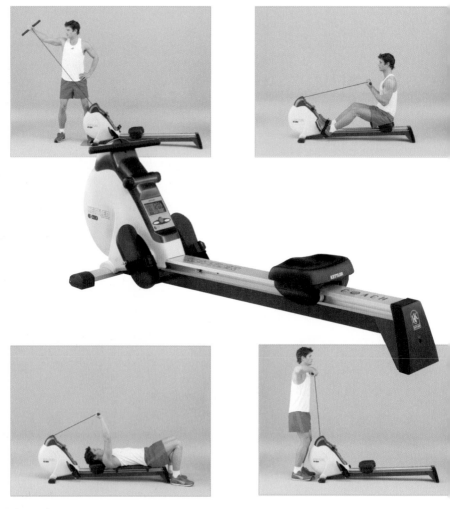

Cross-trainer

The cross-trainer enables effective whole-body training that works all the large muscle groups and boosts the fat metabolism. The cross-trainer is particularly suitable for low-impact conditioning training and for weight reduction. The cross-trainer provides a unique, weightless training feeling due to the innovative elliptical motion path of the foot pedals.

The even movement offers a particularly low impact strengthening of the legs, bottom and hips. The arm action linked with the leg action strengthens the arms, shoulders, chest and back. The larger the flywheel, the more even and low-impact the whole movement.

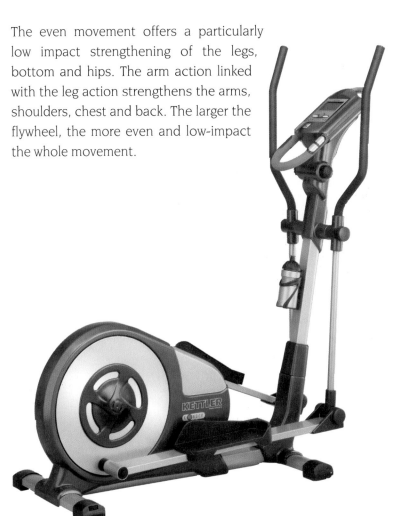

Gym Bicycle

Ergometer bikes and exercise bikes are the classic training equipment for training at home. The circular motion path is easy on all the lower limb joints. Unlike exercise bikes, ergometer bikes are electronic and feature a precise loading control and a very accurate display. Again, the larger the flywheel, the more evenly and quietly the machine runs.

Stepper

The stepper trains the cardiovascular system and the leg and bottom muscles. The product range of the *Kettler* Stepper includes the *mini stepper* with or without computer and with variable traction, such as the *stepper comfort* with hand grip and hand heart rate sensors. Kettler produces a *Power Stepper* with an individually adjustable hydraulic cylinders, stable frames and ergonomic grip.

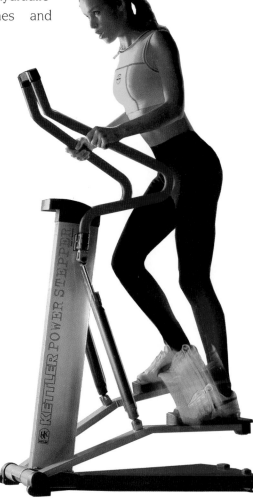

CHAPTER 8

Heart Rate Monitors

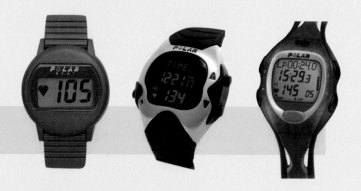

Heart rate measurement has been indispensable in competitive sport for years as a control factor, and since the '90s, wireless heart rate monitors have been used more and more frequently in fitness and recreational sport. This enabled more intensive heart-rate controlled cardio training and heart rate monitoring was integrated more and more into aerobics classes. As a result of the success of Spinning®, the use of heart rate monitors in the gym has become commonplace. The latest research results – translated into new technology (OwnZone® monitor by Polar) – enable simple, individual, sport-specific training monitoring.

8.1 Heart Rate Variability as a new Measuring and Control Factor in cardiovascular Training

Heart Rates – quantitative Heart Work

The heart rate at rest, at sub-maximal and maximal loads and in the recovery phase is connected with loading intensity, loading volume and the efficiency of the cardiovascular system and muscles.

This makes it very useful as a testing and control parameter in endurance sport.

Heart rate measurement can be used for performance diagnosis, load measurement, recovery monitoring and health monitoring.

Heart Rate Variations – qualitative Heart Work

The heart rate per minute gives no information about the length, length difference or the structure of the individual heart phases.

The heart action is subject to great chronological fluctuations at rest and after loading. These are called heart rate variations or heart rate variability, and can be termed the quality work of the heart (readable on an ECG).

For example: In a resting heart rate of 60 beats per minute, theoretically, there must be a heart beat every second (every 1,000 ms). However, in a healthy heart, the rate can fluctuate by milliseconds.

Heart rate variations have been used for a long time in medical diagnosis, for example in cardiology, for risk assessment in cases of heart rhythm disturbance, in pharmacology for testing the effectiveness of cardiovascular medicines or in psychology and occupational medicine for stress diagnosis.

They were first used for training monitoring when Polar 1995 made R-R-Interval (beat-to-beat) recording possible in the Vantage model.

Factors influencing Heart Rate Variation

Heart rate variation is a very "sensitive" parameter. Influences on heart rate variations come from:

▶ The vegetative nervous system
▶ The time of day (circadian rhythm)
▶ Age (high values for children, decreases with age)
▶ Inter-individual differences (genetic influence)
▶ Psychophysical stress, mental tension
▶ Illness
▶ Physical loading

Measurement variations also include loading-heart-rate-related influences, such as work-related stress, infections and fitness level. So, it is possible to determine an individual target zone using these variations.

The Importance of Heart Rate Variation for Training Monitoring

The *OwnZone*® function based on the measurement of heart rate variation during physical activity. It automatically calculates the effective and safe intensity level for training. The personal heart rate target zone is established during a 10-minute warm-up phase.

The *OwnZone*® corresponds to about 65% of the maximal heart rate, and training in the *Own-Zone*® thus enables fitness-oriented training in the aerobic zone.

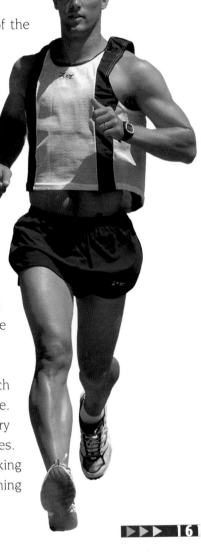

In practical terms, *OwnZone*®/heart rate variation means that it is possible to establish an individual training zone that can vary according to daily form and sport type.

In the warm-up, the heart rate variation is measured in milliseconds on an increasing heart rate. The variability decreases and plateaus at the start of the aerobic training zone (about 65% of the maximal efficiency).

This gives the lower heart rate value, which marks the start of the aerobic training zone. This measuring method can be used in every warm-up and lasts a maximum of 10 minutes. There are courses in *OwnZone*® centers working on this principle and enable individual training monitoring.

8.2 A Range of Heart Rate Monitors

Polar has developed three very different series, each with different heart rate monitors, in the market to cater for all types of athlete:

▶ The Polar A-Series – the introduction could not be simpler
▶ The Polar M-Series – training could not be more personal
▶ The Polar S-Series – train like the pros

The A-Series: for beginning Trainers, Fitness and health-oriented Athletes

Training with a Polar heart rate monitor enables personal fitness and training goals to be reached efficiently, and also leads to an improved general level of physical fitness.

If you want to get fit without suffering unnecessarily, you must train at the correct loading intensity, i.e., neither under nor overload yourself.

The easiest way to control intensity is by the heart rate. Every Polar heart rate monitor consists of a wristband receiver and an ergonomic and, therefore, very comfortable chest belt transmitter.

The M-Series: your personal Fitness Trainer

So, you want to improve your fitness, maybe also lose a few pounds and improve your well-being. Then the Polar M-Series model is the right training partner for you. Based on new measuring technology, this new heart rate monitor automatically determines your own personal training zone, the OwnZone®. Your OwnZone® can vary from day to day, according to your physical and mental state. Your OwnZone® is the optimal training zone for your training on a specific day.

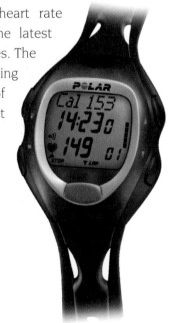

The S-Series: Train like the Pros

Polar presents the next generation of heart rate monitors: a fortuitous combination of the latest training science with innovative technologies. The Polar S-Series launches you into a new training dimension, developed with the aim of defining your training in a new way, making it more individual than before.

Functional Sportswear

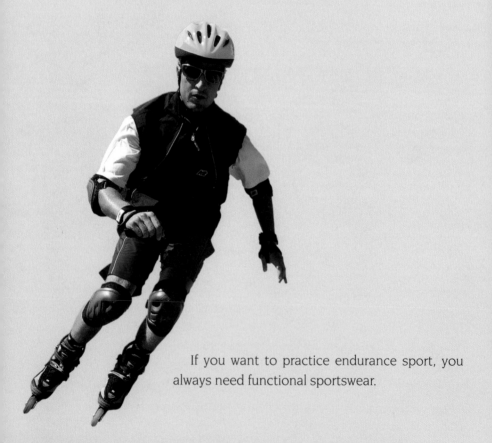

If you want to practice endurance sport, you always need functional sportswear.

Why is functional Sportswear necessary?

?

All healthy exercise implies physical activity during which our bodies work like engines generating energy and heat. Sweat is the natural cooling water that stops the body from overheating. The more energy output generated by physical activity, the greater the amount of sweat produced.

Up to 1.5l of sweat are produced per hour during intensive exercise. The faster and more intensively you move, the higher the energy and heat production will be. But only a third of this heat production is used for performance, the other two-thirds are required by the body in order to regulate its heat balance.

► Physical activity generates energy
► The body converts two-thirds of this into heat
► Only a third is used for sporting performance

Sweat means moisture. Moisture takes heat away from the body, reduces the insulating performance of clothing and causes an unpleasant feeling. Wet and cold clothes are a health risk.

In order to prevent colds, muscle tears and injuries, functional sportswear is necessary to transport the sweat away from the skin. All layers of clothing must be breathable (= permeable for water vapor) so that sweat can evaporate. A waterproof layer is also necessary in order to prevent the permeation of moisture from outside (rain, snow, dew).

Table 27: Advantages of functional sportswear

Functional Sports underwear	Functional Sportswear
▶ Fast sweat transportation	▶ Sweat transport
▶ No danger of colds	▶ Breathable
▶ Optimal efficiency	▶ Isolation against the cold
▶ No unnecessary weight	▶ Cooling effect – due to sweat transportation and breathability (no condensation)
▶ No unpleasant odors	▶ Waterproof – against external moisture
▶ Warm and dry to wear	▶ Windproof – against wind chill factor
	▶ Light weight
	▶ Freedom of movement

The wind chill factor

People find that with increasing wind speed, particularly in winter, the actual temperature is a lot lower than that shown by the thermometer. Meteorologists call this wind-related cold the "wind chill factor."

In simple terms, the wind chill factor works as follows: when the human body produces heat, a thin layer of heat forms around the body, which the wind blows away. The stronger the wind, the thinner the layer of heat, and we begin to freeze. If the worse comes to worst, we get a cold. The table below shows the wind chill factor for different wind speeds.

Tab. 28: The wind chill factor

External temperature	12°C	6°C	0°C
At 10 km/h	10°C	3°C	-4°C
At 20 km/h	6°C	-2°C	-10°C
At 30 km/h	3°C	-5°C	-14°C
At 40 km/h	2°C	-7°C	-16°C

What is the 3-Layer Principle?

To meet the standards of functional sportswear, the firm Loeffler has developed the 3-layer principle (underneath, in-between, on top). The layers must be optimally compatible with each other, so that each layer can fulfill its tasks. Several flexible, thin layers protect better against the cold than one thick layer. A thick layer also limits freedom of movement.

▶ Functional sports underwear, the underneath layer, has the job of transporting the sweat quickly away from the skin, so the skin stays dry. This should prevent the cooling of the body and colds.

▶ The "in-between" layer has the job of keeping the body warm and protecting it from cold. Materials with plenty of trapped air are the most suitable, as air is the best insulator. In the past few years, fleece has established itself for this function. Tights and trousers made of different materials are also suitable.

▶ The "top" layer has the job of protecting from cold, wetness and wind. Many materials offer this protection. If it is a matter of protection from adverse weather, while guaranteeing breathing ability, then only a few materials will do. According to the area of use, there are very different materials available. Colibri, Gore-Ultra-Lite and Gore-XCR-Wear are completely waterproof; Windstopper Activent – Wear is absolutely windproof. Both materials are very breathable and let the sweat evaporate.

Table 29: The 3-Layer principle

3-Layer-Formula	Layer	Materials	Type of clothing
Underneath	Functional underwear	Transtex X-light	Vests Pants
In-between	Warm layer	Fleece Transtex Elastic Coolmax	Shirts Jackets Tights Trousers Jumpsuit
On top	Weather protection	Gore-Tex-XCR Gore-Tex-Ultra-Lite Windstopper/ Activent Colibri	Jackets Blousons Trousers

Training
Tips

Endurance training is ideal for losing weight, as it strongly boosts the energy metabolism at the correct intensity. The training volume can be increased to levels that stimulate the fat metabolism (lipolysis) relatively quickly, i.e., with a loading duration of more than half an hour, and an intensity of 60-70%.

10.1 Endurance Training Basics

In most endurance sports, it is difficult to overtrain. However, you should visit your GP to check for possible heart problems and also check your physical resilience (exercise ECG). Such a health check should be repeated annually.

In particular, all exercise beginners and those with previous illnesses or with risk factors (overweight, diabetes, lack of exercise, high blood pressure, smoking, high blood cholesterol) should consult a doctor before taking up a sporting activity.

Table 30: Training tips for endurance sport

A health check before exercise – first the doctor, then the exercise
▶ Beginners or "returners" over the age of 35
▶ In the case of previous illnesses or complaints
▶ In the case of high risk factors (e.g., overweight, smoking, high blood pressure, high blood cholesterol, diabetes)

No endurance training if you are ill or have a cold
▶ If you have a cough, flu, fever or rheumatic pains, take a break from training
▶ After the break from training, train more lightly (reduce intensity and amount)

Avoid over-training
▶ Start slowly and continuously increase the loading (intensity frequency and duration)
▶ Preferably train under supervision (club, running group, gym)
▶ First, increase the content, then the intensity
▶ Pay attention to how you feel on the day

Recovery
- ▶ Rest is required after training (recovery, sleep)
- ▶ Massage and sauna are also a good idea
- ▶ Schedule a light training session after a heavy one

Preventing and healing injuries
- ▶ Warm-up and cool-down belong to every training session
- ▶ Injuries take time to heal
- ▶ You can always fall back on other sports (cross-training)

Take the prevailing weather conditions into account
- ▶ Functional sportswear (air exchange, heat insulation, windproof, etc.)
- ▶ In hot conditions, reduce training and take in sufficient fluids
- ▶ In high ozone and pollution levels, miss, reduce or postpone training (train in the morning or in the evening)

Take care to eat and drink correctly
- ▶ High carbohydrate, low-fat diet
- ▶ Replace the fluids lost during exercise by drinking mineral water

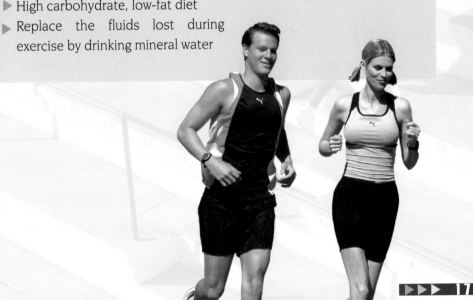

Most people have already started a diet or fasted and then very quickly lost their resolve. Just as many people have taken up a sport with great enthusiasm, only to give up just as quickly feeling frustrated with themselves.

There are different causes, which are, in most cases, avoidable. By observing a few essential, basic rules, even in endurance training, you will stick with it and have fun and success in training and in your goal of losing weight.

Table 31: Avoidance of typical drop-out problems

▶ Realistic goal-setting

▶ Well-planned training program

▶ Regular training

▶ Not too intensive training

▶ Fun and enjoyment in training

▶ Allow yourself a break now and then

▶ Try out different sports

▶ Integrate seasonal sports (e.g., cross-country skiing in winter; inline skating in summer)

10.2 Warming up

The three-phase training session (warm-up, workout, cool-down) is valid for all the endurance sports described.

The duration can vary considerably according to the intended performance level, fitness and health of the individual. Despite the relatively low injury risk of endurance sport, the warm-up is an absolute "must." A specific warm-up program should start every training session.

The Warm-up Effect

The warm-up has many effects. A focused, well-balanced warm-up stimulates the metabolism, which in turn raises the body temperature, activates the cardiovascular and respiratory systems and brings the muscles to be used up to a working temperature.

So, from a physiological point of view, the whole body is prepared for the activity to follow. This firstly reduces the risk of injury, like muscle pulls or soreness, and secondly increases subsequent physical efficiency.

In endurance sport, the warm-up can generally be split into two parts:

> ▶ Gentle running, walking, cycling or swimming to activate the cardiovascular system
> ▶ Stretching the muscles to be used in order to prevent injury and enhance performance

The above order is tried and tested, but in swimming, the stretching is often done first (risk of hypothermia). The loading intensity is low during the warm-up, but should still be gradually increased, even during this phase. The duration of the warm-up should be at least 10-20 minutes, according to the target group and depending on the subsequent loading intensity and the external conditions (e.g. low temperature).

Along with the positive effects of the warm-up on the *physical performance level*, there are also positive effects in the *psychological* and *social* areas. So, for example, a gentle ride on the Spinning® bike, a slow run or a relaxing stretching session increases the mental readiness and motivation for the training to come.

The sportsperson reacquaints himself with the medium once again (e.g., water, snow, type of terrain) and to the equipment (e.g., bike, skis, inline skates) and is motivated for the activity that follows. Participants get to know each other better and get used to each other through communal exercise and during small-talk in the breaks.

To sum up, we can speak of a psycho-physico-social warm-up, where the individual areas mutually influence each other.

Activation of the cardiovascular System

Gentle jogging, walking, cycling or swimming are general warm-up activities. They should always be carried out first, i.e., before stretching, as warmed muscles that are well-supplied with blood can be stretched even better. The intensity is very low (50-60%).

The duration is usually about 3-7 minutes at hobby sport level and up to 15 minutes in competitive level endurance sport. For the less well-trained, alternating the warm-up intensity is recommended in the first months (e.g., for running: 2 mins walking; 1 min jogging; 2 mins walking, etc.).

With time, the jogging proportion can be increased more and more. Shaking out the legs while walking is another way to lighten the ensuing running load.

Stretching of the Muscles to be used

Stretching is part of the warm-up and should always be done after the jogging phase, because the muscles to be stretched are better supplied with blood. One of the major functions of stretching is the prevention of injuries, such as muscle pulls or soreness. Stretching does not just reduce the danger of injury but also means that "the activity that follows can be carried out more fluently, harmoniously and with a higher load".

To carry out a complete stretching program requires a thorough knowledge of this area. Please see the relevant literature.

The following exercises should form a minimal stretching program to be carried out before every training session. The muscles concerned should be stretched until tension is felt and then held for about 8-10 seconds according to subjective feelings, until the tension in the muscle subsides noticeably. As you stretch, bear in mind the following basic principles:

▶ Concentrate on the stretched muscle
▶ Don't bounce, jerk or rock
▶ Continue to breathe calmly
▶ Stretch slowly and continuously
▶ Come out of the stretch slowly
▶ Preferably stretch in a set order (e.g., from top to bottom)
▶ Possible two repetitions

In all the endurance sports described, the large muscle groups of the lower limbs are solicited:

▶ Front thigh muscles (quadriceps)
▶ Hip flexor muscles (iliopsoas)
▶ Rear thigh muscles (biceps femoris)
▶ Adductor muscles (adductor magnus)
▶ Calf muscles (gastrocnemius; soleus)

In addition, swimming, cross-country skiing and aqua jogging use the upper limbs, e.g., the chest and shoulder muscles:

- ▶ Shoulder muscles (deltoids)
- ▶ Rear upper arm muscles (triceps)
- ▶ Chest muscles (pectorals)

Shoulder muscles and rear upper arm muscles

In order to stretch the rear upper arm muscles and the shoulder muscles, the arm is taken as far back as possible behind the head and between the shoulder blades. The elbow is then held by the other hand and slowly pulled to the other side. Try not to hollow your back too much during this exercise.

Chest muscles

Stand near a post, a tree or a wall and lean against it with the arms bent at the elbow. Then turn the head and the free shoulder away from the wall, while the elbows remain on the wall. The shoulder can be brought forward a little to make the exercise more difficult,.

Quadriceps and hip flexor muscles

Stand relaxed, but stably, on one leg. Support yourself with your hand on a wall or a post for better balance. The other hand holds the free foot around the ankle and pulls the lower leg slowly upward as far as possible until the heel touches the bottom. At all costs avoid hollowing the lower back as this strains the abdominal muscles and raises the pelvis.

Hamstring muscles

Stretch the hamstring muscles by standing with one heel about 0.5m in front of the other slightly bent supporting leg. The

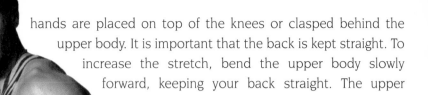

hands are placed on top of the knees or clasped behind the upper body. It is important that the back is kept straight. To increase the stretch, bend the upper body slowly forward, keeping your back straight. The upper body bends from the hips.

Adductor muscles

To stretch the inner upper thigh muscles or adductor muscles, adopt a squatting position with the back as upright as possible and put the soles of the feet together. Place the hands on top of the ankles and try to stretch the inner upper thigh muscles or adductor muscles by pushing them apart with the elbows.

Calf muscles

The starting position of this stretching exercise is wide step of about 0.5 m in front of a wall or a post. The toes are parallel and pointing forward, and the heel of the straight rear leg is pressed firmly onto the floor. As the pelvis is pushed forward, you will feel the tension particularly in the upper calves. If the rear leg is bent slightly, the stretch shifts to the lower calf muscles.

10.3 Cooling down

The *cool-down phase* takes place after the workout, its function being to accelerate recovery, prevent muscle soreness and long-term damage (e.g., muscular imbalance, incorrect posture).

There is a difference between cool-down methods suitable for directly after training and those for some time afterward. Possible cool-down methods are gentle jogging, swimming, cycling or walking, and stretching.

There are other additional cool-down methods, such as aqua relaxation, sauna and psycho-regulation techniques, such as progressive muscle relaxation and autogenic training.

A cool-down (e.g., jog and stretching of the muscles used) should always take place directly after training. The duration of the cool-down depends on the duration and intensity of the preceding workout.

At the recreational level, it should last about 10-15 minutes. At competitive level, it should last at least 15 and up to 30 minutes.

Gentle Jogging, Walking, Swimming or Cycling

They should be deliberate, loose, slow and relaxed. They stimulate the elimination of metabolic waste products (e.g., lactate = lactic acid) from previously utilized muscle tissue, while maintaining a good blood supply to the muscles under low-intensity loading. The duration varies from a few minutes to 10 minutes after very long and intensive loading.

To check the correct loading intensity, you should be able to chat easily while you are jogging, without getting out of breath.

Try to jog so slowly that the heart rate drops continuously. You could alternate between jogging and fast walking. If the loading intensity is still too high, you should walk instead of jog in the cool-down.

Stretching

The most-utilized muscles should be stretched both before and after training. The stretching exercises described above can also be used after training, but the duration of the stretch should be about 20-30 seconds, i.e., considerably longer than in the warm-up.

If there is enough time, the most-used muscles should be stretched a second time. The muscles should also be loosened by shaking them out. The heavily-loaded leg muscles in particular can be shaken out from a relaxed supine position.

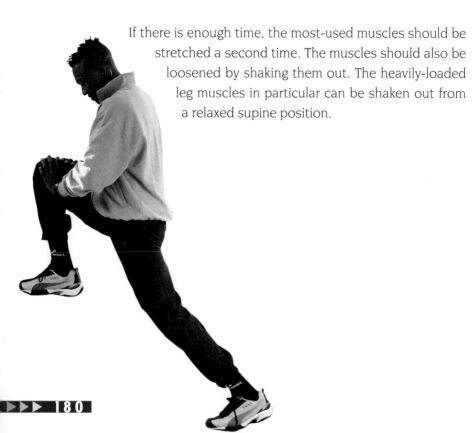

10.4 Cross-Training – motivating fat-burning Alternatives

Who has not experienced the situation in which lack of motivation causes training sessions to be missed or a sporting activity to be dropped altogether? One way of avoiding this problem of motivation is trying other sports and changing sports before you get bored. This is exactly the advantage of cross-training.

There are various possible ways to interpret cross-training:

▶ Seasonal change (e.g., cycling in the spring; inline skating in the summer; walking in autumn; cross-country skiing in winter)
▶ Change the medium or the surface (water, asphalt, sand snow)
▶ Regularly rotate several endurance sports (Tuesdays aqua jogging; Thursdays, Spinning®; hiking during the weekend)

Whether after injury, as injury prevention to avoid overloading, but also on holiday or to increase your own motivation, there are many reasons for "cross-training" in fat-burning oriented endurance sport.

These reasons are by no means just physical. Particulary on the psycho-social level, there are many reasons for mixing endurance sports on a daily basis to make training more varied, attractive and, above all, motivating.

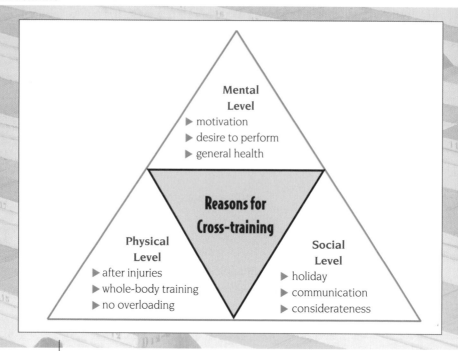

Figure 11: Physical, mental and social reasons for cross-training

Training Alternatives for psychological Reasons

If you often start training sessions feeling completely demotivated, you should look about for suitable alternatives that you want to do, which are not too difficult to incorporate into your daily training routine. Initially, you should not carry out the alternative sports as additional training sessions.

If you normally run three times a week, but suddenly feel like doing aqua jogging, swimming or cycling, do this once a week and eliminate one running session. Over the long term, this does not increase the motivation to run, but leads to better general health and a higher mental and physical desire to exercise.

Training Alternatives for physical Reasons

Typical injuries and complaints (e.g., muscle cramps, shin splints, Achilles tendon inflammation) after regular training are usually caused by the following:

▶ Increasing training volume too fast
▶ Training volume too high (over-training)
▶ No stretching or strengthening exercises of the relevant muscle groups
▶ Bad technique

Many overloading injuries can be avoided by using cross-training as an injury prevention measure. But if it is too late and a small injury has been sustained, rest is not necessarily the only answer. In the case of certain problems or after certain injuries, it is perhaps better to avoid running or cross-country skiing, but you can fall back on alternatives, such as Spinning®, cycling, swimming or aqua jogging, as long as they are not contraindicated on medical grounds. This means that training for weight reduction need not be interrupted during the rehabilitation process. By changing to other sports, strength endurance can even be improved, thereby preventing other future injuries.

A further advantage from the physical point of view is that doing a variety of endurance sports ensures that the whole body is trained. A runner or an inline skater who has hitherto only worked relatively one-sidedly on the legs now also trains trunk (abdominal and back muscles), upper body (chest and shoulder muscles) and the upper limb muscles for example by cross-country skiing, swimming or aqua jogging. Training the above muscle groups also has a positive effect on the metabolism and, by extension, on calorie consumption.

Training Alternatives for social Reasons

There are also many social reasons for varying your endurance exercise program and combining different types of endurance exercise. Exercising with your partner sometimes requires a change of sport.

So, especially when you are on holiday when you are able to spend a lot of time together, you can turn to other sports. Maybe you don't just want to use exercise to boost calorie consumption, but also want to meet other training partners and think you can do this better in group activities, such as Spinning® and aerobics than by running or swimming.

Appendices

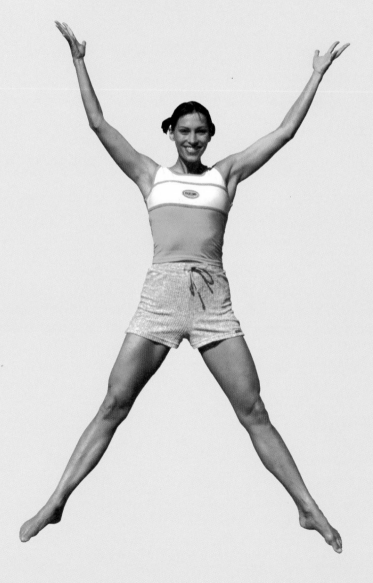

1 Nutrition Lexicon

Important nutritional and training science technical terms are explained below.

Active Metabolic Rate: The amount of energy required daily by our bodies to do work.

Amino Acids: The building blocks of all proteins.

Aspartame: A sweetener that is about 200 times sweeter than household sugar.

Basal Metabolic Rate: The amount of energy required daily to maintain vital bodily functions (breathing, heartbeat, gland function).

Body Mass Index (BMI): Measurement for evaluating body weight.

Bread Unit (US):

Carbohydrate Exchange (UK): Unit for evaluating the glycaemic index of food. Corresponds to about 12-15g of carbohydrate.

Broca formula: Older, now controversial, formula for calculating normal weight.

Caffeine: Active ingredient in coffee beans, tea, cola nuts, mate and (in low quantities) in cocoa beans. Caffeine has a bracing, stimulating effect.

Calorie (abbrev. cal): Now outdated unit of energy (still very common).

Carbohydrate: The third main nutrient group along with fats and proteins. Carbohydrates provide energy and are used in small quantities as building material for the body.

Cardiovascular Diseases: Pathological changes in the heart and/or coronary arteries.

Cholesterol: A fat-like substance needed to form hormones and vitamin D. A too-high cholesterol level in the blood encourages the development of cardiovascular disease.

Coronary: Relating to the heart-supplying blood vessel (coronary vessel).

Depot Fat: The body's fat reserves. Depot fat is used as an energy reserve, a protective cushion for sensitive organs, such as the kidneys and also as a heat insulator.

Diabetes Mellitus: Diabetes; a disorder of the carbohydrate metabolism.

Electrolyte Balance: All physical process affecting the metabolism of minerals. The electrolyte balance is closely connected with the water balance.

Empty Calories: Term for foodstuffs that are very high in calories but contain few or no essential nutrients, such as vitamins and minerals (e.g., sugar and alcohol).

Energy Content (Calorific Value): The amount of energy (in calories or joules). Different main nutrient groups have different calorific values: carbohydrate 4 kcal/g, protein 4 kcal/g and fat 9 kcal/g.

Energy Need: The energy need is expressed in calories or joules and is divided into basal need (basal metabolic rate) and active need (active metabolic rate).

Energy Consumption: Consumption of energy by the body's metabolic processes, breathing, heart beat, movement, etc. Energy consumption depends on age, height, weight, gender and physical activity.

Fibre: Certain vegetable nutrients (e.g., cellulose) that cannot be digested by the human body.

Fluor, Fluoride: Trace element that helps bone stability and hardens tooth enamel.

Folic Acid: Water-soluble vitamin belonging to the B vitamin family. Folic acid deficiencies are common in young people, young women and the elderly.

Fruit sugar (fructose): A simple sugar, mainly found in fruit and honey. Together with dextrose (glucose), it forms household sugar (saccharose).

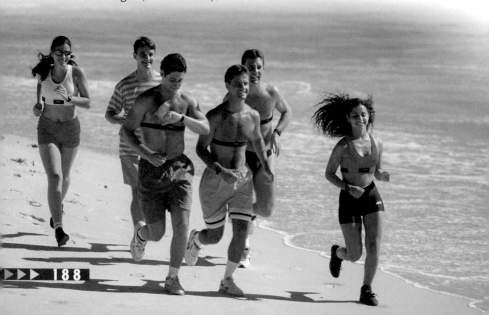

Hidden Fat: Amount of fat in food that is not visible. Meat, sausage, cheese and chocolates in particular contain a high proportion of hidden fat.

Hypertension (High Blood Pressure): Favored by being overweight, high sodium intake, lack of exercise, smoking and stress.

Hypervitaminosis: Health problems caused by excessive vitamin intake.

Infarction: An infarction (e.g., heart attack, stroke) occurs after the blocking of an artery by a blood clot, particularly when the arteries are already blocked.

Joule (abbrev. J): Internationally used unit of measurement for energy. In 1978, the official unit the calorie was replaced by the official unit the Joule. One calorie is equivalent to 4,184 Joules.

Main Nutrient Groups: These include carbohydrates, fats and proteins. They provide energy for the body and building blocks to form the body's substances.

Metabolism: The body's metabolism encompasses all anabolic, katabolic and conversion processes. It maintains body substances and body functions.

Nutritional Value Tables: All the important ingredients of our daily diet listed in table form. The amounts relate to 100g of the food concerned.

Osteoporosis: Bone thinning or decalcification.

Protein: One of the main nutrition groups along with carbohydrates and fats.

Risk Factors: Factors that favor the development of disease, for example, smoking, lack of physical exercise, bad diet and stress.

Raw Vegetables: Uncooked edible vegetarian food, rich in fiber, minerals and vitamins.

Sugar: Term for all sweet-tasting carbohydrates. This term is commonly used for household sugar (saccharose) in particular.

2 Internet Links

▶ http://www.polarusa.com
▶ http://www.polar-uk.com/index.html
▶ http://www.kettler.co.uk

3   Photo & Illustration Credits

Cover photos:
Front – Jump Photo agency; Back top – Polar Electro; Back bottom – Johannes Roschinsky.

Photos:

Engelberg-Titlis Tourism: pp. 123, 144, 146, 150.
Jump: pp. 3, 29, 39, 60, 185.
K2 Sport: pp. 107, 108, 110, 112, 114, 164.
Kettler: pp. 151, 153 left, 154, 155, 156 right, 157.
MPK: pp. 133, 134, 136, 139, 142.
Polar Electro: pp. 7, 8, 10, 25, 36, 37, 46, 51, 55, 57, 58, 62, 67, 72, 75, 79, 83, 84, 88, 90, 92, 94, 96, 97, 100, 102, 103, 105, 106, 117, 119, 121, 122, 124, 132, 143, 152, 153 right, 156 left, 158, 159, 161, 162, 163, 169, 171, 175, 178, 180, 189.
Johannes Roschinsky: p. 9
Sportsphotography Bongarts: pp. 125, 129.
Tecnica USA: pp. 17, 22, 31, 68, 81, 173.
Cover design:
Jens Vogelsang